SPOT ON:

NUTRITION

A holistic strategy for optimal health and performance

Andrew Johnston

CHEK 4, HLC 3, USAT 1

Former professional cyclist and current Ironman triathlete, RAAM finisher, leukemia survivor, and twice voted one of the "100 Best Trainers in America" by *Men's Journal*

with foreword by Paul Chek

NUTRITION

The doctor of the future will no longer treat the human frame with drugs, but rather will cure and prevent disease with nutrition.
~Thomas Edison

WARNING - DISCLAIMER

The workouts and other health/performance-related practices described in this document were developed by the author through extensive study and personal/professional experience. These programs may not be suitable for everyone. Thus, all individuals, especially those suffering from any disease or orthopedic dysfunction, should first consult their physician before undertaking any of the activities or recommendations as set forth in the following pages. The author has been painstaking in his research. However, he is neither responsible nor liable for any harm or injury resulting from the exercises or lifestyle changes described herein.

Published by Triumph Training, 659 Auburn Ave, Ste 201, Atlanta, Georgia 30312, 404 431 2287
Andrew@triumphtraining.com

ISBN: 13: 9781515108498
Printed in the United States of America
Book Design: www.adkinsconsult.com. Photo images: www.dollarphotoclub.com

TABLE OF CONTENTS

FOREWORD

When Andrew asked me if I'd like to write the foreword to his new book, *Spot On: Nutrition*, I said enthusiastically, "It would be my honor!" As a man with thousands of students worldwide and more than thirty years experience teaching and coaching many people through their health crises', I can assure you that it isn't hard to recognize *mastery in the making*. Andrew Johnston is such a man.

Andrew began studying holistic health and corrective, high-performance exercise with me almost fifteen years ago. Andrew has completed my CHEK Practitioner training, which is four years of intensive training on corrective exercise and performance conditioning. He has also completed my comprehensive three-level Holistic Lifestyle Coaching program. Furthermore, he has taken many additional advanced courses and completed those trainings with me personally.

When I first met Andrew, the man who stood before me was lean, strong, extremely fit, and aware—a triathlete with the focus of an eagle. When he shared that he was battling leukemia, it was hard to believe that the guy standing in front of me could be dealing with such a health challenge. *Great Spirit has a wicked sense of humor, and illness is a wonderful teacher!*

The challenge of leukemia would (and does) flatten most people, but not Andrew. Like Biblical Job, he was willing to wrestle with God. Andrew took leukemia's challenge head-to-head; he studied, and diligently applied and practiced all that I have taught him about holistic health, nutrition, and exercise, as well as mastering the teachings of many other fine teachers. He went on to complete another Ironman (six of them) along with other grueling, athletic events and today is a happy, healthy father and business owner.

Over the years that Andrew was my student, we formed a powerful friendship of mutual respect. I've been able to visit Andrew and see his studio in Atlanta. It looked just like him—clean, well-organized, and highly functional. I'm sharing my observations of Andrew because whenever we hold a book in our hand—regardless of the title or how many initials there are behind the author's name—without knowing the author personally, there's really no way to tell whether or not they are a true master, or just a well trained parrot (that types). Consider the fact that there are thousands upon thousands of diet and health books in the marketplace, yet we are still the sickest people the planet has ever seen. Show up at a nutrition conference, and chances are good that many of the nutrition "experts" will be overweight or obese.

Spot On: Nutrition is a practical, highly informative book created for your benefit by a man that has personal and professional integrity inside and out. **He is a former professional cyclist and current Ironman triathlete, RAAM finisher, leukemia survivor, and twice voted one of the "100 Best Trainers in America" by** *Men's Journal.* As we say in the country, "that boy's serious potatoes!" As we'd say in the locker room, "that dude's got balls!" And if you ask me what I think of Andrew Johnston, I'd say, "That man has *wholeness—he's a wise man.*" That's what makes this book so special. Andrew is the living embodiment of the teachings he offers here, a true master, and I can guarantee it!

The Simplest Things Are Most True

In this book, *Spot On: Nutrition*, Andrew follows my footsteps by explaining the simple truths of food, and its basic elements (carbs, fats, and proteins). What Andrew has done better than I have in my books is to provide a well-rounded critical review of the modern thinking that led us away from the truths we once lived. I feel this is particularly valuable to those with the academic mind-set of our day. It is also important if you've "believed" what you read in books, magazines, or learned about on T.V. Andrew isn't on the payroll of a multi-billion dollar a year corporation selling gimmicks as (scientific) truth. His only motivation in writing this book is to use "good science" and clinical experience to explain the shortcomings of "for purchase/sale science."

Though the medical profession likes to tout that "we are living longer (because of modern medicine)," the fact is that we aren't *living longer* as healthy vibrant people; we are just *dying more slowly!* The famous nutritionist, Biodynamic farmer, and pioneering biochemist Erinfried Pfiffer stated in one of his lectures in 1957, "Most people are dead by the age of 35, *and their corpses just keep walking around for another 35 years!*" I think that this summarizes the majority of people around the world as evidenced by the increase in the use of medical drugs by all ages to manage lifestyle issues related to poor diet and nutrition.

Pharmaceutical manufactures, which are as intimate with the medical industry as lovers in wedlock, bolster their pockets with BILLIONS of dollars each year. They have created drugs *for every symptom you are going to experience* (eating and living the way they suggest) *from the time you are born until the moment you die!* My comments shouldn't be interpreted as that I'm suggesting modern drugs and medicine are useless; there is a time and a place for everything. I tell my students, there is no such thing as a bad drug or exercise, only an *incorrectly prescribed drug or exercise.*

Modern medicine (and nutrition) shouldn't really be seen as "curative," for it is actually a highly profitable system of *illness and disease management*—just like a glove fits a hand. Very little of what modern medicine or modern nutrition offers has anything to do with addressing the causative factors of disease. To actually address the causes of what ails most people and manifests as fatigue, obesity, illness, and disease would require modern medical science to "come clean" on the chemical industry, food processing industry, the modern exercise industry, the pharmaceutical industry, the commercial farming industry, and many more! When you reflect upon the taxable income generated by the medical industry alone, to reveal the truth and teach people the simple truths they've forgotten could be considered a national security threat by many governments in the world today. Without all that taxable income, who would fund the military industrial complex?

When we look closely—as I have for the past decades—at what causes the majority of fatigue, illness, and disease, it almost always boils down to this: **avoidance of and/or ignorance of the essential basics of healthy eating and living**. When sick people worldwide consult me for my help with every kind of disease, diagnosis, and life crisis you can imagine; when I look deeply into what is actually *causing* their symptoms and diseases, I commonly find any combination of the following factors:

- Not having a dream bigger than the crisis at hand coupled with a dominance of negative, fear-based thinking
- Dysfunctional breathing patterns
- Lack of sleep and deep rest
- Poor quality food and suppression of one's natural biological instincts to seek, and eat foods in proportions for *their individual needs*
- Poor hydration and the consumption of poor quality (often very toxic) water; a significant number of people today don't even drink water—only processed beverages
- A lack of exercise (or movement) in general; among athletes, the challenge of over-exercising is more common.

Like Andrew, I don't "fix people." I teach my students and my clients how to love, respect, and care for themselves. I teach them that caring for their body requires meeting their basic needs effectively, just as caring for plants or pets does. Andrew and I both firmly believe that when one invests the time and energy to "create health," there is no place disease can exist! If you are going to spend your time, energy, and resources on yourself, it seems logical to invest in and create health each day. Particularly when you consider being ignorant or passive with your health and well-being means your investments flow "out of the family circle" and into big industry, while your quality of life diminishes day-by-day.

When we consider the often quoted (but seldom adhered to dictum) *"you are what you eat!"* as an unavoidable reality, knowing how to eat correctly becomes paramount. If we examine the profound effects nutrition has on our biochemistry, and how our biochemistry dramatically affects our physiology, especially our hormones, which in turn affects our psychology—our thinking and our moods—learning to eat optimally and ideally for your individual needs turns out to be the difference between living well and *being a corpse walking around waiting to die.*

As a humanity, we are at a critical time in our history when we are being called to be the very best we can be so we can better care for the planet, our families, and our communities. As I often say to my clients, "if you can't do it for yourself, do it for your children and for the world."

This well-written, informative book by Andrew Johnston—a true master of all aspects of nutrition, exercise, and holistic living—focuses on the nutritional component of what ails people at large. If you want to think clearly, feel vital and energetic, be creative in your life, look good, have great sex, and enjoy a *quality* life, then this book is ideally suited for you! When we eat and live with respect for our food; when we support sustainable farmers and corporations that offer only wholesome, natural foods and products, we support *earth friendly* practices we can all enjoy. We recover a piece of our humanity. And we cultivate a legacy for those that follow.

> **Love and chi,**
> **Paul Chek, HHP**
> **Founder, C.H.E.K. Institute**
> **Founder, PPS Success Mastery Program**

ACKNOWLEDGMENTS

The performance of the human body is dependent on a variety of nutrients. How a book performs in the marketplace is not much different as a daunting array of factors must come together for the final product to be truly ready. In the course of writing this book, I've enlisted the aid of countless people—all of them serving as micronutrients working synergistically to nourish my creative desires until they were healthy enough to be shared. This book would never have been possible without them.

In the acknowledgments of my first book, *Holistic Strength Training for Triathlon*, I credited Paul Chek as being my co-author. I honestly cannot think of much I do during any given day which is not somehow impacted by Paul and everything he teaches at the CHEK Institute. After graduating from his program (though not his influence), I was tasked with writing a thesis to obtain the level of Master CHEK Practitioner. One page turned into several, and weeks passed into months. When it was complete, I realized it wasn't finished. Health never is. Thus, the thesis evolved into this book. Yet, when you're discussing the Foundational Factors of Health, how do you decide when to write the final paragraph? Maybe another one of Paul's students can pick up where I left off, but I believe *Spot On* is a good start. And I thank you, Paul, for this along with all the other beginnings you have given me.

Dodie Anderson and Dan Hellman should share the next mention. Dan is a mentor who ultimately became a colleague and good friend. His selfless guidance eventually led me to Dodie who took my understanding of nutrition to the next level—and the level beyond that. She has an uncanny way of making the complex accessible and would likely have made a much better author for this book. But I don't think she enjoys the limelight. Maybe when you've got it, there's simply no need to flaunt it. Someone needs to give her props, though. She's helped hundreds of people take control of their health, including me. For that reason I'm more than honored to put what she's taught me on paper so a larger audience can benefit from her expertise.

I also need to thank Matt Cole of Podium Multisport. I knew I had another book in me. But the success of my first book is what gave me the confidence to even think about a second one. Matt has sold more of my books than Amazon, I bet. To compliment the best bike fit in the business, he has his customers buy and then implement the concepts in *Holistic Strength Training for Triathlon*. Guess he got tired of people breaking down before their bikes did. One thing's for sure—Matt's constantly looking for ways to improve the services he provides. That he thinks enough of my work to promote it near and far means a lot to me.

Numerous clients had health issues which forced me to expand my professional tool box. And while some may never know they served as the impetus to take a specific class or read a particular study, all of them should know working with them is what gave me the skills and authority to write any of my books. Two clients, specifically, I recruited to read various parts of this text. Dave Siereveld is a friend and—more importantly—a retired English teacher. Julie Seaman is another friend and client who developed a keen interest in nutrition (my ego likes to believe it was because of my influence, of course). She's a professor of law at a local university and took time from her busy schedule to lend a critical eye to this Nutrition section of *Spot On*. If my writing could hold up under their scrutiny, I knew my editor's red pen would gather a bit more dust. Additionally, various friends on Facebook read and commented on a few "teaser" chapters I posted on my page. I used a lot of their suggestions (and had to de-friend only a couple of folks in the process...).

The universe introduced me to Robbie Adkins. She's the creative genius who made this book more than a simple Microsoft Word document. While that feat may not have stretched her capabilities, the back-and-forth of designing the cover with me probably tested her more than when she could have ever expected when she first agreed to be my graphic designer. I'm hopeful any stress I caused her severely impacts her short-term memory—as I'm asking her to format all the other books in the *Spot On* series coming out soon.

Finally, as I did in my first book, I want to say a last thank you to my family. My son renewed my interest in health from the first moment I held him. Life became instantly more precious as I welcomed him into the world, fiercely holding him and his mom in a tearful embrace. I cherish the duty of their care, even though I know it's a responsibility only they can truly take for themselves. More than anybody then, this book is for them. My son made me, in a sense, immortal. And my wife helped make an infinity worth living.

INTRODUCTION

Time doesn't stop—even if you do.

That thought was stronger than the stench of urine as I sat cramping in a hot, dark port-o-let about ten miles short of the finish line of the Great Floridian Triathlon. Somewhere outside, my comfortable lead was quickly becoming less comfortable as second and third place inevitably hunted me down. I could hear other triathletes running past, calling for water or coke or Gatorade. The aid station was in full gear. The volunteers handed out everything from bananas to chicken broth. And even though I doubted they had any muscle relaxers, it couldn't hurt to ask, right?

But first I had to get off the toilet seat.

I tried again to stand and the flurry of contractions riddled my legs like gunfire. The confines of my private bathroom were making the cramps worse. The heat of the Clermont sun was concentrated in the port-o-let. And last I looked, the finish line wasn't in here. I needed to get outside again. Putting my hand on the only thing I could without contorting into a position that would illicit another cramp, I grabbed onto the lip of the urinal and pulled my body up. My quads twinged, but I was out the door and moving before I could even question again why I was doing another Ironman.

Like most goals in life, my motivation was multifaceted. But I think the main reason I was in Florida suffering through 140.6 miles with my fellow masochists from all parts of the globe can be traced to a statement I made in a moment of bravado: "Don't worry about me, I'm gonna be the first Leukemia Survivor to win the overall of an Ironman." And I don't really know who I was trying to convince—myself—or my family and friends who were watching me slowly deteriorate after a diagnosis of Chronic Myelogenous Leukemia. But the constant fear and sadness reflected in their eyes was more palpable than the pain that haunted my bones, and I couldn't begin to heal until that look changed. They had to believe I was going to be okay. They had to trust that I was going to be around for a while. Dying's the easy part. We all do it sooner or later. It's going on that's hard sometimes. Bound by a memory is no different than being tied to an I.V. So I gave them all hope by making a promise I wasn't really sure I could keep.

But today I was trying.

The race began well before the horn sounded to start the swim. And if you're reading this, you probably know much of my story. So I'll just pick up at the end of lap one of the swim. I looked at my watch and saw thirty-one minutes and change. And even though I had an official in a kayak redirect me back on course since the chop of the water made it hard to navigate, I knew I had been swimming well. The course must be long. Well, no worries. Everyone has to swim it. So I trudged up to shore, unable to high step due to cramping in extreme range of motions, and started the second lap one minute down on first place. The next lap was a little straighter, and I exited the water in 1:03— my slowest Ironman swim ever. Strippers (not the kind on the poles) helped me with my wetsuit or I would've had to ride 112 in neoprene—rear delts locked up every time I tried to reach the zipper. Running into the changing tent, I saw the leader headed out of T1. You better ride fast, my friend...

Once on the bike, I'm at home. I've spent over half my life racing bicycles, and I've gotten pretty good at pushing pedals. The Parlee I'm riding this year is the best bike I've ever owned. And while my skills on two wheels peaked several years ago, technology has helped me retain some sense of speed. Put me on something like my Parlee, and I feel confident enough to ride with anybody. This was a race, however. And I could tell from the first pedal strokes that the sleep loss over the past few weeks was affecting me. It took me 30mins to take back the two minutes the leader had on me heading onto the bike course. But with a century and a marathon still to go in the race, I was doing what I said I'd do over eight years ago: I was winning the Great Floridian.

Other than a wrong turn on lap two when a cop directed me back onto lap one, the bike was fairly uneventful. I was frustrated with the fatigue I felt during my time to shine but hoped my lackadaisical pacing would be rewarded on the run. Besides, even on a bad day, I'm not going too slow—I just hope it's fast enough to have the gap I'll need for the run. Somehow that discipline has improved to where it's slowly becoming my strength. Crazy for me to say that, as I still don't consider myself a runner. The Kenyans aren't exactly what you would describe as short and stocky. But I don't run scared anymore. I know I can hold off my competitors. But can I hold off the cramps...?

I rolled into T2 where I left off on the swim—slowest Ironman bike ever—5:28. But feeling about the same as before the ride was a good sign. As I ran out to start the marathon I wondered how much of a buffer I'd have for the marathon. "You have 5 or 10 minutes!" someone yelled. "I'd be happier with more!" I responded. Just then, a cyclist rolled up to escort the leader, and I got a nice pump knowing the leader was me. I felt good—the hints of cramps in my quads were there, but they seemed to be sinking deeper and deeper below the surface with each step I took. The first mile went by in 6:40, and I consciously tried to slow down. The second mile included a pee stop in a port-o-let which would become too familiar a couple of hours later. But it was still a 6:55. "Slow it down, Drew," I told myself. And finally I settled into a pace between 7:30 and 8:00, a pace I felt comfortable with and which allowed me to answer the questions of my escort. It was kinda like we were out for a stroll, and the conversation eventually turned to why I was out there. I told him about my promise, and he showed me the yellow Livestrong band on his wrist he wore as a *Survivor* of prostate cancer. He wondered aloud if he should take it off with all the Lance crap coming out. I didn't answer him. That decision was his.

I set the time on my watch at the first turnaround to see how much time I had on second place. I kept expecting to see him as the seconds crept slowly by. But it took a while before we saw each other. I analyzed his form as we got closer. He looked good. But as we passed each other, I looked at my watch—over nine minutes. I've got at least eighteen on him with twenty to go. Was that enough? How fast was he running? I'd have to wait till the next turnaround to find out.

At the second turnaround, we repeated the game. Second still looked good, but this time I had twenty-two minutes on him. I'm faster. And with less than eighteen to go, the surreal feeling of leading an Ironman was beginning to—a knife in my right quad, and I immediately stop. My guide rolls on ahead, completely oblivious that cramps have left me frozen on a hot piece of Florida tarmac. I've cramped at every race I've done since starting chemo, so I'm not too worried. I immediately start doing the math of runs and splits as I try to will the quads to relax—I should stretch them. But I know that lifting my heel to my butt will make the hamstrings catch, and I'd like to keep my rigamortis to a minimum. If second is doing eight minute miles, and I'm not moving...I try walking, but each extension of my knee turns the leg to stone. I close my eyes and breathe into my belly, calming myself. I take the time to sip some water and get some calories into me. And when the muscles relax into tiny, sporadic shivers, I risk moving forward again. The twinges are still there, but they stay just below the surface as I run at a much reduced pace to go find my escort on his bike.

A mile later I make it down a hill without cramping only to be rewarded by both legs locking up. My guide is with me now and asks if I need some water. I tell him I'm on chemo, and this is just one of the unfortunate side effects— especially if you're an endurance athlete. Yawns will cause my face to cramp. Brushing my teeth causes my hands to cramp. I've even had one day on the bike when I waited too long to go pee, and my cremaster muscle cramped. And for those of you reading this who don't know your anatomy, consider yourself lucky.

The marathon becomes a series of spurts and stops as I can't make it through a mile before cramps overtake me. My legs alternate between stiff and stone, and when not running I must look like I'm posing in a bodybuilding contest. Immobilized while trying to leave an aid station, I hear a girl say "look at his calves!"

I somehow get moving again, but now the cramps are moving up to my upper body. I have to put my gel flask in my singlet—my fingers keep fixing in unnatural positions, alternating between modified versions of thumbs up, hang ten, and F-You! Gotta relax my grip, cause I don't want to piss off the locals. And I continually need to straighten my arms as the brachioradialis on both sides won't let me bend them. But the worst are the muscles in my head and neck which force me into jaw gymnastics trying to release them. I'm nearing the water stop half way up a hill that roughly marks the 10K to go point. The course is filled with competitors on this last lap, yet I feel more alone than ever. I'm shuffling more than running now, and I realize this race has turned into a death march for me. Then a brutal barrage of cramping stops even that.

I've cramped every day of my life since starting Gleevec. But I've had more days of life because of Gleevec than many who came before me. Yeah, I have a lot to be thankful for. I think of Team in Training. I think of my doc at Atlanta Cancer Care. The images of friends come as fast as the contractions firing off in my legs, and I look around at the triathletes who run or walk by. I've attracted the attention of the volunteers at the aid station who come down the hill with offers of gels and ice. When I don't move, they ask if I need help. My eyes close. Silently, I retreat into my own thoughts as I shake my head so they know I heard them, that I'm lucid. I think about the friends and family who make up my support group and wonder what news they're able to get on-line or via phone calls or texts. Are my boys at Podium Multisport cheering my victory unaware that I might not make the finish line? Are Diana and Declan back at transition, getting the announcement that the leader has stopped. With my eyes closed, I see second place pass me for the lead as I stand petrified in the middle of the road just half a mile from an imaginary finish. The same finish I've dreamed about for eight years. And win or not, I just want to cross that line. But the seven miles of asphalt which lie between me and it seem impossible. I'd crawl if I could. But I can't.

So I run.

Somehow I run. I convince myself to stop running like I'm going to cramp. Quit being tentative and run with my normal stride, unrestrained and through a full range of motion. Forward progress doesn't come easy. The actin and myosin fibers in my legs have been glued together for so long now that any movement feels like I'm tearing them apart. And I probably am. And I'm probably going to be more sore tomorrow than I've ever been in my life. But I'm moving. Slowly at first as I climb up the hill to the turnaround. And as I start my descent, I'm torn between the gift of gravity and the pain of impact as my feet hit the ground harder. Yet, with each stride, I'm gaining momentum. I'm gaining confidence and feel for the first time in several miles that I can actually pull this thing off.

A runner I'm not sure I recognize passes me going in the opposite direction looking strong. Could that be the new second place? I check my watch. It's been a little over three minutes since I hit the turnaround. I've got less than seven minutes with six miles to go. God don't let me cramp. I run through *the twenty-first mile in 8:30. I see the guy who had been in second place a few minutes later and run the next mile at about 8:20. Making sure I grab nutrition, I run through the aid stations, afraid that stopping might stop me. Congratulations are now coming from people who recognize me as the leader. "Bring it home!" they say, or something similar—I don't really hear them despite my thumbs up acknowledgement. I'm half focused on form and half focused on the crazy possibility that I'm not cramping even though every stride is testing that belief.*

Somewhere in transition the site of Declan jumping up and down stirs me back to consciousness. I automatically reach down to give him five but pass him and Diana before the thought even registers. I almost turn around but don't want to risk stopping. The guy behind me is probably gaining. And I'm sure my body can't sprint now. At the final turn around, I hear "you got this" and finally begin to believe it's true. The smile I usually wear when racing—my testimony to anybody watching that I'm still alive, that I appreciate the blessing of being healthy enough to compete—makes a belated return to my face, and I realize I'm really going to win. The sign directing runners onto laps two and three or the finish is ahead, and I joyfully head in the direction of my name being called over the P.A. I slow to a walk a few feet from the line and throw my hands in the air. I almost don't want this moment to be over. Yet, just across the line I can see the race clock ticking.

Time never stops in an Ironman.

And neither do I.

Now, that's not exactly the introduction I had envisioned when I decided to write this book. It may not be what you thought you'd read either. Perhaps you expected something a bit more technical—paragraphs filled with impressive jargon which made for difficult reading yet gave me an air of authority. After all, we're talking about complex issues here. Psychology. The Autonomic Nervous System. Sports Nutrition. To discuss these subjects with any credibility, the letters PhD have to appear after your name. And if you dare to write anything worth reading or studying or even changing a lifestyle, you better bring something other than your credentials to the discussion.

You better bring the truth.

Well...unfortunately, the truth really hasn't been a prerequisite in *any* field of science lately. Maybe that's because too much research is bought and paid for. These days, the Financial Agenda often corrupts the Scientific Model.

In *Tainted Truth*, Cynthia Crossen points out the suspicious correlation between the results of "research" and the financial interests of its sponsors. For example, Dr. Richard Davidson reviewed 107 published studies and could not find a *single case* where a drug/treatment manufactured by the sponsoring company was found to be inferior to another protocol. Without resorting to outright fraud, the researchers can obtain these miraculous results by adjusting the length of the study, manipulating dosage levels, and various other questionable practices. If those techniques aren't sufficient, however, *then* fraud is a pretty good backup plan. From a COPE statement made on the inappropriate manipulation of peer review processes:

> *The Committee on Publication Ethics (COPE) has become aware of systematic, inappropriate attempts to manipulate the peer review processes of several journals across different publishers. These manipulations appear to have been orchestrated by a number of third party agencies offering services to authors. This statement is issued on behalf of COPE after consultation with a variety of publishers to underscore the seriousness with which we take these issues and our determination to address them.*

> *While there are a number of well-established reputable agencies offering manuscript-preparation services to authors, investigations at several journals suggests that some agencies are selling services, ranging from authorship of pre-written manuscripts to providing fabricated contact details for peer reviewers during the submission process and then supplying reviews from these fabricated addresses. Some of these peer reviewer accounts have the names of seemingly real researchers but with email addresses that differ from those from their institutions or associated with their previous publications, others appear to be completely fictitious*

> *We are unclear how far authors of the submitted manuscripts are aware that the reviewer names and email addresses provided by these agencies are fraudulent. However, given the seriousness and potential scale of the investigation findings, we believe that the scientific integrity of manuscripts submitted via these agencies is significantly undermined.*

Money is the motivation. Drummon Rennie, in the book, *Trust Us, We're Experts*, states that *"Universities and scientists are seduced by industry funding and are frightened that if they don't go along with gag orders, the money will go to less rigorous institutions."* And *The Ecologist* reports that only 75 out of more than 15,000 drug and food chemical researchers could be considered independent. The others? Their pockets are being lined with industry dollars at the cost of your health.

Another reason the truth is so difficult to find is that for any one study which "proves" black, you can find two which argue white. What's going on here? Perhaps it's our definition of authority which has changed. We place more stock in celebrity than we do science. And if we recognize a face, we'll likely buy into a belief—even if it doesn't serve us.

Yet, that's **exactly** how you know when you've found the truth—**when it works for you**. As Zen Master Thich Nhat Hanh writes:

A teacher cannot give you the truth.
The truth is already in you. You only need to open yourself -body, mind and heart-
so that his or her teachings will penetrate your own seeds of understanding and enlightenment.
If you let the words enter you, the soil and the seeds will do the rest of the work.

My race report from the 2012 Great Floridian is the culmination of what works for me. And while it offers you only a glimpse of my mental and physical preparation, this guide is going to take you much deeper. My goal with this writing is for you to realize that health and performance are synonymous. One can not exist without the other—not for long. And the fact is, for most of us, the event we train our entire life for *is* life. So whether you're an Ironman or an Everyman, you are an athlete—one who needs to be prepared for the demands of your chosen sport as well as the life you choose.

It's not the fastest who wins.
It's the one who slows down the least.

Most of an athlete's race performance is predicated on life outside of competition. After all, racing is a stress. But if you stress a system which is already in the red, you risk breaking that system. Thus, the basis for athletic success is built upon sound nutrition and lifestyle principles that allow a competitor to endure the demands of training and make it to the competition healthy.

Of course, I know what some of you might be thinking. *"But didn't you have leukemia? That's not exactly healthy!"* And whether you're playing devil's advocate or you're just an inquisitive pain in the ass, that's a valid point. So, let me address those comments right here, right now:

I *have* leukemia. I will always have it. And though it may be difficult for some to appreciate this concept, leukemia has become a good teacher for me.

See, there was a time when I couldn't cross the finish line truly happy unless I came in first. But if you see any of the pictures of me from the Hawaii Ironman, you'll see I had a smile on my face the whole day (bawling in my wife's arms after the race doesn't count). I was ecstatic to just toe the line. To get another chance to pursue a passion. To achieve a goal. To test myself against myself. Yes, I have leukemia. But leukemia doesn't have me.

I was healthier than anybody on the start line of The Great Floridian. Fact is—I'm healthier than just about anybody you'll ever meet. Admittedly, that's not much of a boast these days. I've studied some of the premiere experts across a variety of fields. And, unlike a lot of talking heads, I'm not just an academic. I won't claim to *know* anything until I've experienced it myself. After all, you can study all you want about how to ride a bike. But until you've tested your equilibrium against the force of gravity, I suggest you keep your training wheels on.

I *know* health because I *live* health.

On race day, none of my competitors stood a chance. I had visualized winning The Great Floridian so many times that first place was already mine. The 140.6 miles which stood between me and the top step of the podium were just a formality. My fueling strategy during the event—while right on target—really didn't matter much either. My everyday nutrition had set the table for race day success. And my training, despite being limited due to the demands of job and family (as well as a keen understanding of the possible detriments of excessive endurance development), was specifically programmed to eliminate any potential weaknesses while delivering me to the starting line in top condition. Indeed, every possible nutrition and lifestyle principle was working in my favor.

And now they can work for you.

With discussions running 180 degrees opposite of conventional dogma, I'll explain how *all* of the body's systems are interconnected. The reductionist approach to science has done nothing but reduce most of us to lesser beings, far from our potential. In the pages of this guide, you'll realize how the cumulative impact of *EVERYTHING* you do—how you think; how you eat; how you sleep, breathe, and more—how each one of these daily activities impacts your performance. Good or bad, it all adds up.

Regardless of the arena, a focus on the *Whole* is what lays the groundwork for champions to be made; from which vitality can thrive. It doesn't really matter how hard you train. It's not even a question of taking the right pill or employing the latest technology. When we fail to merge *simple* with *science* and approach the body from a holistic perspective, we are literally off-center. Constantly looking for the edge, we instead find a dangerous precipice. Our foothold on the foundation of health becomes unsure. Storms of misinformation swirl around us, continuously threatening our balance. And once we lose our equilibrium, we also lose sight of the truth.

The following pages will help you regain that perspective. I wrote this book to assist you in finally discovering what's possible...for *you*. And if by some chance you somehow managed to stay grounded in the middle of the chaos that claimed far too many others, the contents of this book will help solidify your position on health— make it unshakable. You won't ever have to call it a comeback if you never lose it. You simply have to stay *spot on*.

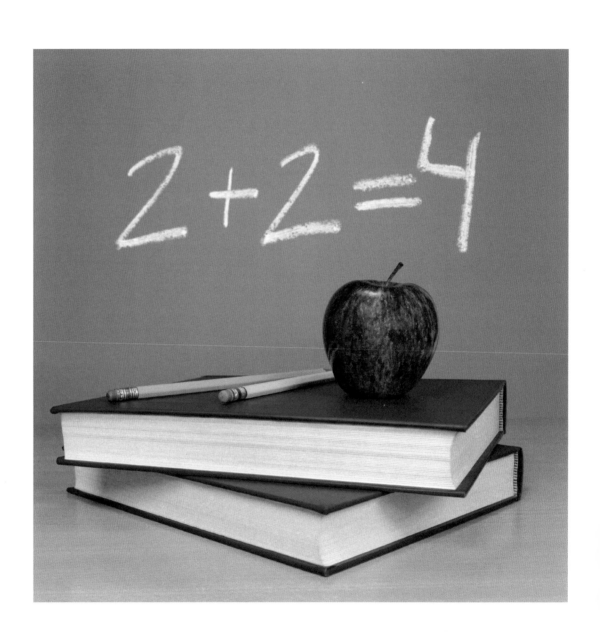

CHAPTER ONE

Keep it simple, stupid!
—lots of folks

Here's the main dish. And since I know we all have different tastes, I'm gonna try and serve this section up in a few different ways. So depending on your appetite, you may find you've had your fill after the first course. Simple and without much flair, this chapter will likely be what many of you have been craving. But for those of you with a taste for something a bit more complex, the remainder of this section will tantalize your palate and allow you to heap as much information on your plate as you can stomach. Even so, my advice is to start small. Take each offering and chew it over thoughtfully. Give yourself a chance to truly digest every piece you take in so it can be assimilated into knowledge—that's a critical nutrient lacking from the Standard American Diet (S.A.D). And the deficiencies inherent to ignorance are costing us more than our health. So if you're hungry and have a hankering for a hearty portion of truth, I invite you to dig in.

- Food that's healthy generally doesn't need to tell you how many calories it contains
- The more ingredients in a food, the worse it is for you.
- The longer the shelf life of a food, the worse it is for you (the exceptions to the rule are raw seeds/nuts and fermented foods like sauerkraut).
- The more health claims made about a food, the worse it is for you.
- If you can't pronounce an ingredient in a food, don't eat it.
- If it hasn't been on this earth for 5000+ years, don't eat it.
- If it won't keep your dog alive, don't eat it.
- Don't put it in your mouth if you don't know where it's been.
- If it came from a plant, eat it. If it was made in a plant, don't.
- Stay away from HYDROGENATED/PARTIALLY HYDROGENATED foods (baked goods are a major culprit).
- Stay away from ARTIFICIAL COLORS/SWEETENERS/FLAVORS or PRESERVATIVES (just about anything pre-packaged).
- Eat organic/local—it's better for you, the environment, and the economy.
- Eat a balance of macronutrients (carbohydrate/fat/protein) at every meal/snack.
- As a general rule, color is a proxy for nutrient density in a food. If it's the color of cardboard (e.g., cereal), it probably has about the same nutritional value.

Did you enjoy that? Good! Wipe your face, and you may be excused now.

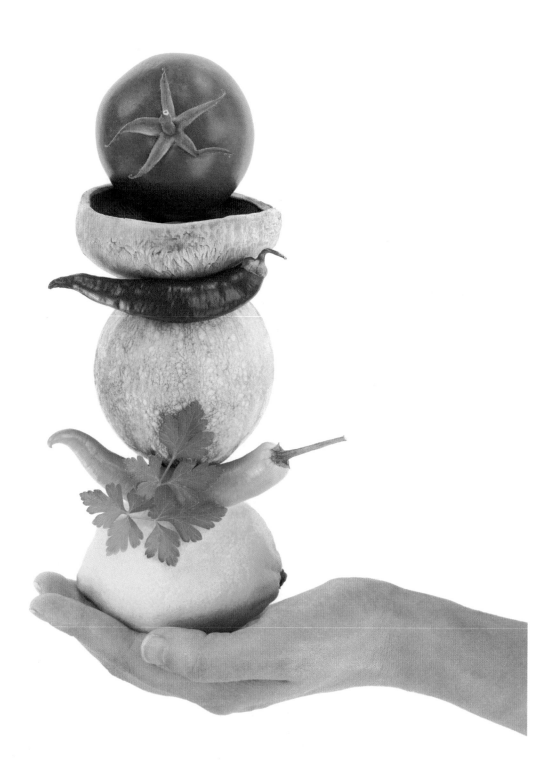

CHAPTER TWO

Food is an important part of a balanced diet.

—Fran Lebowitz

Are you ready for seconds?

I hope so, because I've been slaving away all day. And if you've read this far, you're probably salivating by now. Well, you've come to the right place: I'm serving up info you can use to satiate a ravenous desire for health. So, if you're hungry for knowledge, there's a whole lot more where that came from!

Yet with so much to choose from, you might be wondering what to put on your plate first. Well, not to brag or anything, but you really can't go wrong with anything I'm offering—it's all good. If you want a suggestion, however, might I recommend you start with the macronutrients?

Some of you reading this may think I'm just trying to stir the pot. After all, can you think of a subject more polarizing than carbohydrates, fats, or protein? Depending on whom you ask, each of these macronutrients typically falls somewhere between Mother Teresa and the Anti-Christ. People can be so dogmatic in their allegiance to a particular diet it's like trying to talk politics or even religion. But once people realize there's no such thing as a bad macronutrient—just bad approaches to macronutrient consumption—we can go a long way towards healing our bodies and our views of what constitutes a healthy diet.

Let's first consider carbohydrates. And when I say carbohydrates, please notice I did not spell it *G-R-A-I-N-S*. A lot of foods other than breads, cereals, and pasta occupy this category: any fruit; any vegetable; basically anything which doesn't have the ability to protect itself from human consumption belongs in this group (though you'll eventually see that these foods aren't quite as defenseless as they appear...). Dairy and honey along with sugar and other sweeteners also qualify as carbohydrates.

The reason most of us can't think outside the box when it comes to defining carbs probably stems from the USDA's infamous food pyramid. The brain child of a woman named Luise Light, the original diagram included a base composed of fruits and vegetables. By the time her idea was introduced to the American people, however, the Grain Lobby had "*convinced*" the USDA that the bottom of the pyramid should be built on 6-11 servings of bread, cereal, rice, and pasta. And don't ask me why corn wasn't included. Guess its reps must have been out of D.C. that day....Either way, Ms. Light criticized the move, saying

...the health consequences of encouraging the public to eat so much refined grain, which the body processes like sugar, was frightening! But our exhortations to the political heads of the agency fell on deaf ears. The new food guide, replacing the 'Basic Four,' would be a promotional tool to get the public to buy and consume more calories, sugar and starch.

Grains are in the Bible for God's sake, so I really don't know why Ms. Light got her panties in such a wad! Cereal—pasta—our daily bread—it's all good for you. Just ask any grain farmer. Or talk to a baker. Better yet, consult with any registered dietician whose higher education was funded by General Mills or Quaker Oats or any of the other Big Food...Conglomerates

...the big...food conglomerates ...the big...food...

Oh.

I see—the best way to market a product or service is to convince consumers it's good for them. Throw in a few closed door meetings to negotiate the government's stamp of approval, and buyers will come in herds! Soon the sheeple will be so sick, fat, and complacent that it's hard to tell where the conventionally raised cattle begin and the grain-fed masses end.

Hmmm.....maybe Ms. Light did have a beef.

Either way, that's at least part of how grains became synonymous with carbohydrate. And maybe that's why so many other carbs ended up with such a bad rap. Guilt by association, I suppose. But the truth is, there's nothing wrong with carbohydrate.

Carbohydrate is to the body what gasoline is to a car. And just as there are different types of gas, carbs, too, fall into different categories: monosaccharides, disaccharides, and polysaccharides.

- **Monosaccharide**—one sugar molecule (e.g., fructose, galactose)
- **Disaccharide**—two sugar molecules (e.g., lactose, sucrose)
- **Polysaccharide**—long chains of simple sugar molecules (e.g., glycogen, starch)

Notice that each of the definitions above uses the term *sugar* in the description. That's because all three types of carbohydrate break down into glucose in the body—that is, if they're broken down at all. Some polysaccharides are considered indigestible. Cellulose, for example, cannot be broken down by any organism lacking cellulase. And if you're human (no offense, cause I've been called that at times, too), you don't possess this particular enzyme. But, hopefully, you *do* have a highlighter as you might want to remember this particular fact—it will prove important, later during the course of our discussion on nutrition.

So carbohydrates, in general, break down into sugar (glucose) and are delivered to the cell to be used as fuel. Thus, it's safe to say the body's preferred source of energy is glucose. Ray Peat, a pioneer in nutrition and physiology since the early 1970's writes that sugar is the primary source of energy from the beginning of an animal's life.

That's a keen observation. However, some people might argue that an infant learns to crawl before it learns to walk. Thus, maybe fat oxidation is a skill which takes time to master. After all, it's clearly more efficient. Each gram of fat contains nine calories compared to the meager four calories supplied by one gram of carbohydrate. And even the leanest of athletes has enough fat stores to run a marathon without putting much of a dent in the body's supply. Indeed, many competitors spend years training themselves to become fat burning machines in an effort to increase performance.

But could this approach be counter productive?

Older people are better at metabolizing fat than sugar. So are diabetics. Even overweight people, believe it or not, are pretty good at burning fat compared to their ability to use carbohydrate. Yet most competitive athletes I know aren't aspiring to be fat geriatrics with blood sugar handling problems.

Sorry about that: my ability to go off on tangents rivals that of my high school geometry teacher. Let's return to the subject of this chapter. And lest some of you accuse me of fat bashing, I want to go on the record that nothing could be further from the truth—fat's actually one of my top three macronutrients.

It's ironic to me that most people think of fats as either "good" or "bad", "healthy" or "not healthy". The ones naturally occurring in our food, in fact, actually belong to the classification of lipids known as "neutral" fats. Composed of fatty acids and glycerol in a 3:1 ratio (thus the name triglyceride), neutral fats are either solid or liquid at a given temperature dependent on the length of their fatty acid chains and their degree of saturation.

saturated fatty acid

unsaturated fatty acid

double bond

- **Saturated**—carbon bonds are full or saturated with hydrogen atoms and, thus, no double bonds (e.g., butter, coconut oil)
- **Monounsaturated**—one double bond (e.g., olive oil, macadamia nut)
- **Polyunsaturated**—two or more double bonds (e.g., corn oil, soy oil)

Note that nothing in nature occurs in isolation. Just as a combination of micro and macronutrients will be present in any dietary source, all three types of fat mentioned above will be found together in a particular food. For example, coconut oil is 92.1% saturated fat. The remainder is made up of a monounsaturated fat called oleic acid (6.2%) and a polyunsaturated fat called linoleic (1.6%). That's right. Just like any other foundational factor of heath, *real* nutrition is always holistic.

Unlike carbohydrate, which is used almost exclusively for energy, fat has many critical functions in the body. It's a storage site for fuel when more calories are consumed than immediately necessary. And while not of obvious importance in a society where drive through windows and 24-hour convenience stores abound, the ability to store energy has been paramount for human survival. Indeed, one of the reasons we are here is because our ancestors possessed a genetic ability to survive in times when food was scarce.

Fat ensures our survival in other ways, too. It acts as an insulator, protecting the internal organs and other structures of the body as well as helping prevent heat loss. Yeah, you may hate those love handles now. But back when we were cave men and women, they were all the rage. You might want to keep that in mind for when the next Ice Age rolls around.

As a nutrient, fat is commonly found with protein which helps us segue into the introduction of this final macronutrient. That's right—now we're getting down to the meat of the chapter. Or the eggs or the dairy; or even the beans of the chapter if that's your preference. And while I'll try not to play favorites (as talking about barbecue ribs or king crab legs for the next page or so wasn't my plan), there are differences in proteins which need to be addressed. As the second most abundant molecule in the human body after water, quality and source should be of the utmost importance. After all, not all protein is created equal.

As omnivores, humans have an uncanny ability to survive off a wide variety of different diets. Too many of us, of course, have allowed financial or political agendas to influence our dietary practices such that we're testing the definition of the prefix *omni*. But there are two criteria any protein should meet for it to be considered a viable source for human nutrition: bioavailability and "*completeness.*"

Bioavailability

Protein is a constituent of each one of our cells. And not just *our* cells. Every living creature—from insects to livestock to plants—is made up of protein. Thus, every living creature is a potential source for the protein we require. But just because something has protein doesn't mean you can access it or do anything with it. Often the protein is tightly bound up in cellulose and meager human digestion isn't adequate for its extraction. That's one reason you can't eat grass. You're not a ruminant herbivore. You don't have multiple stomachs. You don't spit your food back up and chew the curd (I hope).

You need a middle man to help make some proteins available for human use. Sometimes that middle man is a cow. And sometimes it's the protein manufacturers who use technology to do what the human body can't (or shouldn't). Either way, for the sake of simplicity, let's focus on some of the more common sources of protein in the human diet. Consider the following image:

Protein Source	Bio-Availability Index
Whey Protein Isolate Blends	100-159
Whey Concentrate	104
Whole Egg	100
Cow's Milk	91
Egg White	88
Fish	83
Beef	80
Chicken	79
Casein	77
Rice	74
Soy	59
Wheat	54
Beans	49
Peanuts	43

A couple of man-made concoctions have somehow beaten out whole eggs for the top spot on the Bioavailability Index. Maybe I'm just not an overachiever; or maybe I'm too much of a momma's boy. Either way, I'm gonna trust Mother Nature on this one. 100% is good enough for me.

At the other end of the spectrum is the humble peanut, with a score of 43. Of course, the list above is by no means an exhaustive one, so George Washington Carver can rest easy—the crop he's credited for making so popular is higher than many other foods in regards to the bioavailability of its protein.

Complete Protein vs. Incomplete Protein

The other critical factor in protein choice is dependent on the amino acid profile. All proteins are made from amino acids. And though there are some 500 different types, there are twenty-two common ones. Of these, nine are considered essential.

histidine*
isoleucine
leucine
lysine
methionine
phenylalanine
threonine
tryptophan
valine

Histidine was once considered an essential amino acid only in infants. However, studies demonstrate that a deficiency in histidine is associated with a failure of normal erythropoiesis (red blood cell production).

Unable to synthesize these amino acids at levels sufficient to maintain health, the body must acquire them via the diet. Foods which contain all nine are typically derived from animal sources, though some plant based sources exist as well (e.g., soy beans—but before you order a tofurkey for Thanksgiving, I suggest you read the chapter on soy beginning on p. 75). However, incomplete proteins can be combined in the diet so that the amino acid profile is considered complete. Think rice and beans. Rice is deficient in lysine, and beans are lacking methionine. But the two compliment each other. Indeed, the more romantic of my readers might say these two foods complete each other.

God, that's cheesy!

And perhaps combining specific foods to make a complete protein is a lame nutritional strategy, too. If you look at the bioavailability of both rice and beans, you'll see they score 74 and 49 respectively—well below the standard set by a whole egg. Thus, when pairing incomplete proteins, the health conscious match maker needs to be aware that codependent relationships can often be dysfunctional....

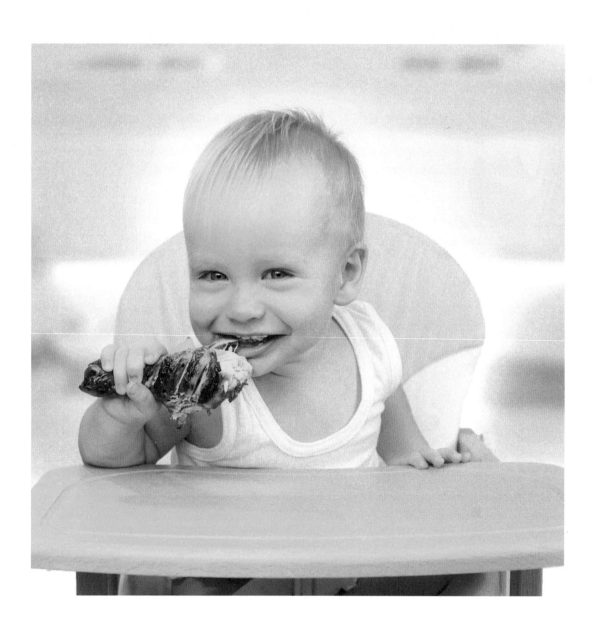

CHAPTER THREE

A man loves the meat in his youth that he cannot endure in his age.

—William Shakespeare

Now that the macronutrients have all been introduced, let's get to know each of them a bit better—starting where we left off with protein. It's arguably the most versatile of the three macronutrients. Providing the basic building material for the body, protein has become almost sacred among gym rats across the country. But to limit the discussion of protein's role in the body to its structural function would be like picking a trainer because he has a nice body. If the trainer is educated, he'll be able to design a program tailored for you. And if *you're* smart, it's the trainer's brain rather than his brawn which will get you to hire him.

Likewise, protein is more than just muscle. It's also the connective tissue—your ligaments and tendons. It's the enzymes like amylase or pepsin or any of the other biological molecules essential for almost any biochemical reaction in the body. Protein is critical to healing. Protein's critical for repair. It helps in the transport of substances like lipids or even oxygen. Your immune antibodies are a type of protein. So is growth hormone and insulin. Basically, protein is everything!

Geez...I'm starting to sound like a body builder.

But I'm not one. Nor do I eat like one. In fact, it's the focus on muscle that has gotten plenty of meat heads in trouble—both in the gym and in the kitchen. For a more thorough discussion on the pitfalls of training the muscle rather than the movement, I invite my readers to explore the pages of *Holistic Strength Training for Triathlon*. For now let's concentrate on the detriments to health when the proteins in the diet become too muscle bound.

Muscle meats like beef or chicken or pork tend to be high in tryptophan. Since tryptophan is one of the essential amino acids, you could assume that more is better. However, when reflecting back on the first two sections of *Spot On*, you may have started to pick up on a theme: *there's a lesson in less*. The more perceptive of my readers might have extrapolated an even deeper truth from those earlier pages: *health is found in homeostasis*. Quiet the mind and discover yourself. Slow the breathing to find health. And when talking nutrition, <u>equilibrium is likewise the state from which vitality can best be explored.</u>

11

It wasn't that long ago that we used to eat the whole animal. And I'm not just talking about your grandmother's liver and onions. I'm talking about bone broths. I'm talking about soups and stocks made from oxtail and chicken necks. I even had a teacher in elementary school who claimed to love fish eyeballs! But now most of us would call that gross...well, really, eyeball consumption was gross back then, too. Either way, today we waste the majority of the animal. Yet by doing so we throw away a lot of valuable nutrition. And we unwittingly throw the amino acid profile of our diet out of balance as well.

Tryptophan is necessary to all forms of life. Research shows that depriving young animals of tryptophan increases mortality, so I think its status as essential is well earned. Yet that very same research demonstrates that feeding older animals a diet deficient in tryptophan actually *increased* longevity.

What's going on here?

It could be that after a certain age, we're not growing so much as repairing. And just about anything—including an essential nutrient—can be the trigger for a multitude of problems when consumption outpaces need; especially if that need changes, right?

Of course, I wouldn't jump to any conclusions. The landing may not be what you expect. But I do think it's fair to ask if perhaps some of the so-called *"non-essential"* amino acids become increasingly important as we get older. Maybe tryptophan should stop hogging the spotlight of the American diet and let other amino acids have a turn at center stage. Specifically, allowing glycine and proline to headline a little more often would help our performance along with our health.

It could be pointed out that a dietary source for glycine or proline isn't even necessary because our bodies can actually synthesize these amino acids. And while I hate to be the purveyor of a *"yeah, but"*, that argument doesn't take into account the fact that excessive tryptophan can actually impair glycine receptors in the brain. Other studies show that tryptophan and some of its derivatives can interfere with the amino acid proline, too.

Can't we just consume more glycine and proline? I know of a health food store right beside the burger joint—there's got to be a supplement or something we can take.

Well, that's one approach—albeit, an ineffective one. See, it's a little like addressing postural aberrations in the body. You don't simply strengthen the long, weak, or inhibited muscle. You really need to stretch the short, tight, or facilitated one at the same time. Otherwise, the system remains unbalanced. Likewise, you don't just add a dietary source of glycine and proline. You also need to reduce the amount of tryptophan in the diet. And cutting back on muscle meats is a good place to start.

Now, I probably lost quite a few of you with that last line. But, please, bear with me. Yes, minimizing muscle meats is a good strategy to start balancing out the amino acid profile in your diet. Despite what some of you may think, though, I am most definitely *not* advocating veganism or vegetarianism or any other manifestation of *"ism"*. I'm quite simply too attached to my bacon—and my health (and that's a whole other can of soy worms which we'll have to save for later). The truth is that grains, nuts, and seeds are all high in tryptophan, too. So eschewing meat is no better than chewing meat. Yet before you smugly chalk up one for the carnivores, let me give you your RDA of reality: the majority of poultry and livestock in this country are fed a diet of grains. Thus, eating conventionally raised meat is like asking tryptophan for a curtain call. And, unfortunately, an encore of this amino acid comes at a cost.

That price, as always, is our health. A review appearing in the 2003 edition of *Immunology and Cell Biology* reads that "*a clear association has been made between tryptophan catabolism and inflammatory reactions in a vast array of disease states.*"

Cancer may be the most costly. At the very least, it's typically the one which makes us pay attention. Research shows that tryptophan catabolism suppresses anti-tumor immune responses. However, I will admit a large majority of these studies are performed on rats. Thus, even though we're talking the Big C, you still may not be too invested. More than a few gerbils met their demise while in the care of people just like you, so how resilient can rodents be? Where are all the studies using human subjects?

Go to the mall.

That's right—just go to the mall. I know it's not a scientific laboratory. Still, if you take a trip to the nearest shopping center, especially during a holiday, you'll see a pretty accurate representation of our current state of health. Lord knows you don't have to be a medical researcher to look around and realize we're not doing all that well. But for those of you who'd prefer a more objective analysis, consider the following statistic as it appeared in an issue of *The Oncologist*:

1 in 2

That's the number of men predicted to get cancer in the U.S as reported by the Surveillance Epidemiology and End Results (SEER) program at the National Cancer Institute (NCI). The prediction for women, sadly, is not much better. It's 1 in 3. And I really can't figure out what's more pathetic—those stats or that our health is so shitty there's a big enough audience for a publication entitled *The Oncologist*. The researchers conclude that these numbers will double by the year 2050, due in part to an aging population.

A population that's not growing so much as repairing maybe....

Of course, these troubling statistics cannot all be attributed to the consumption of tryptophan. Some of the effect likely comes from the displacement of glycine.

13

Glycine

The smallest of the 20 common amino acids, glycine aids in detoxification and stimulates gastric acid production. Low stomach acid inhibits digestion which both impairs nutrient delivery and also decreases energy production. That should make you think twice about taking antacids for heartburn. Indeed, many people on antacid medications (up to 90% by some estimates) actually don't have *enough* hydrochloric acid. Regardless, neither impaired nutrient delivery nor deficient energy production is conducive to maintaining a healthy body. The latter especially will be a recurring theme throughout this book and sets up what I call a Seesaw of Sickness:

When Energy Production goes down, Adrenaline goes up.
When Adrenaline goes up, Intestinal Circulation (of glucose and O$_2$) goes down.
When Intestinal Circulation goes down, Endotoxin Production goes up.
When Endotoxin Production goes up, Liver Function goes down.

Speaking of liver function, glycine also plays a critical role in the detoxification system. It's one of the key nutrients required for efficient Phase 2 Detoxification by the liver, primarily via the amino acid conjugation pathway. When glycine is deficient, this second stage slows, the liver becomes overloaded, and a variety of harmful substances begin to accumulate in the body:

- contaminants
- drugs
- food additives
- pesticides/insecticides
- micro organisms

Most of these substances are fat soluble and end up in adipose tissue or other fatty parts of the body, including the brain. Many of these chemicals are carcinogenic as well. Even hormones and the numerous end products of the body's own metabolism can become toxic when left unchecked. Prolonged, systematic exposure results in a continual down regulation of the various metabolic processes in the body, which are essential for optimal functioning and health. Thus, building on the seesaw example above, a more thorough explanation would look like this:

*When **Energy Production** goes down, **Adrenaline** goes up.*
*When **Adrenaline** goes up, **Intestinal Circulation** (of glucose and O$_2$) goes down.*
*When **Intestinal Circulation** goes down, **Endotoxin Production** goes up.*
*When **Endotoxin Production** goes up, **Liver Function** goes down.*
*When **Liver Function** goes down, **Toxic Load** goes up.*
*When **Toxic Load** goes up, **Energy Production** goes down.**

And then the process starts all over again...

*__*The terms in bold will be intimately explored in Chapter Nine__*

But like all seesaws, if you're not enjoying this ride, all you have to do is get off. Simply return to a more traditional diet. No, you don't need to go out and fill your plate with fish eyeballs (though I guarantee you corneas would be a better staple in your diet than corn). But a food rich in glycine would help balance out your proteins. Specifically, I'd recommend adding some gelatin.

Gelatin is made from all the "*left overs*" of an animal—the collagen, the bones, the gristle—basically the connective tissue. As such, it's void in tryptophan. It also has relatively low amounts of the other amino acids, like histidine and methionine, that are readily found in all the muscle meats. In place of these essential amino acids, gelatin supplies a good dose of amino acids considered to be "*conditionally essential.*"

One of those conditions, of course, would be the desire to remain healthy. And gelatin helps you do just that by providing plenty of glycine. You also get a significant amount of proline. The most vital function of this amino acid is arguably in the maintenance of quality skin—your biggest organ of detoxification (weighing approximately 10% of your body weight). It's also essential in the formation of collagen and other connective tissue so you can move pain free. Gelatin is a good source for alanine, too. This is another nutrient which assists in the elimination of toxins. Additionally, it helps maintain glucose levels and, thus, energy production in the body. In short, gelatin is exactly what you need to stop the Seesaw of Sickness.

But if there's one thing I know, it's never just one thing. As Ray Peat says:

> While some of the toxic effects of an excess of individual amino acids have been investigated, and some of the protective or harmful interactions resulting from changing the ratios of the amino acids have been observed, the fact that there are about 20 amino acids in our normal diet means that there is an enormous number of possibilities for harmful or beneficial interactions.

Humans are complex creatures. We are an integrated system of systems in which is summated every experience we've ever had, nutritional or otherwise. Thus, it's not the specific nutrient which dictates the state of a particular organism. It's the state of the cell which dictates the response the organism will have to whatever stimulus is encountered. From a nutritional perspective, there's more to health than protein and amino acids. And so we don't make the mistake of taking the reductionist approach to health, might I suggest we expand this discussion to other nutrients?

Loosen your belts, ladies and gentlemen. It's time to chew the fat.

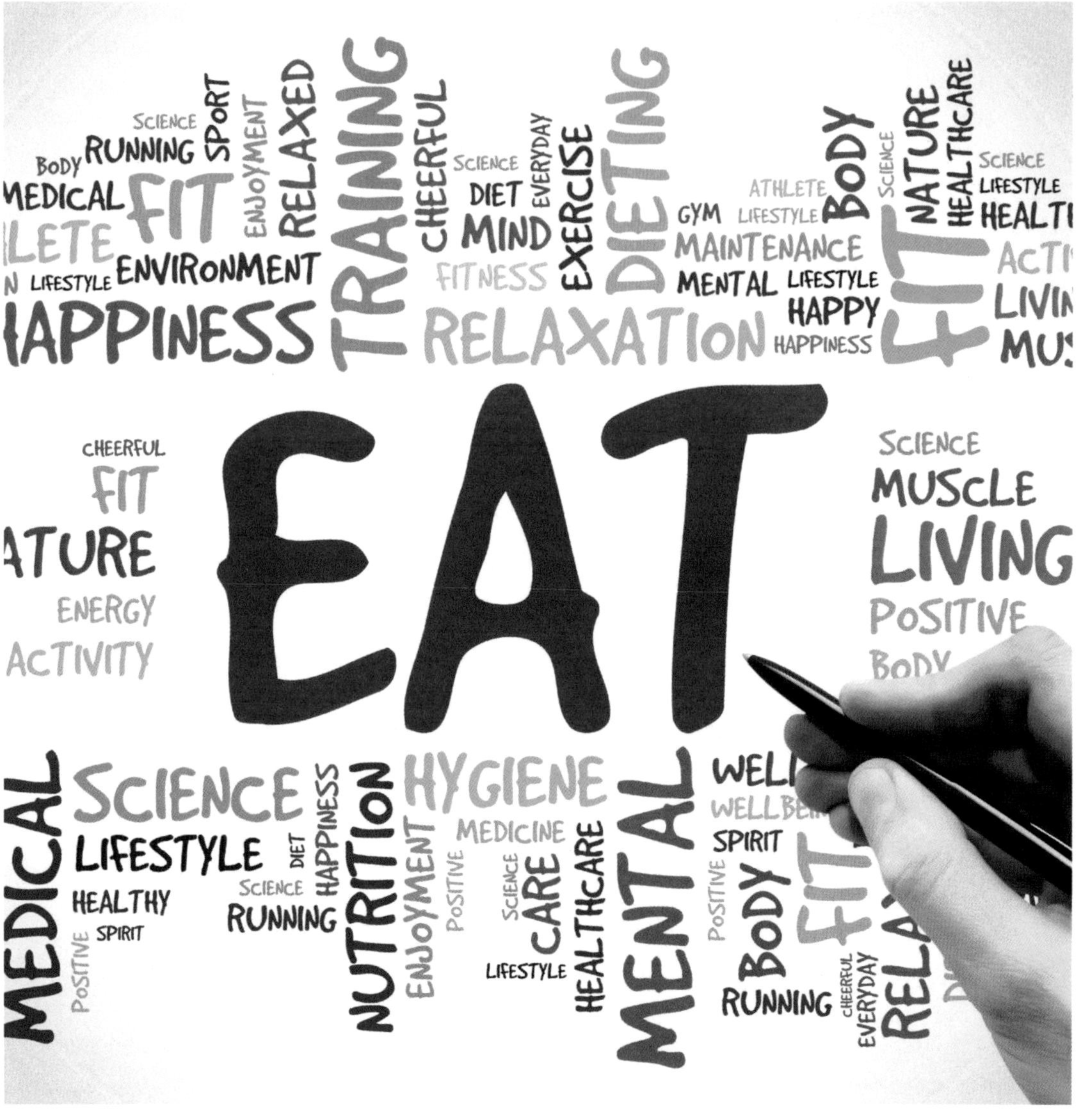
EAT
SCIENCE
SPORT
BODY
RUNNING
MEDICAL
FIT
ENJOYMENT
RELAXED
TRAINING
CHEERFUL
EVERYDAY
DIET
MIND
EXERCISE
DIETING
ATHLETE
GYM
LIFESTYLE
MAINTENANCE
NATURE
HEALTHCARE
ENVIRONMENT
FITNESS
MENTAL
HAPPY
HAPPINESS
RELAXATION
MUSCLE
LIVING
POSITIVE
ENERGY
ACTIVITY
HYGIENE
MEDICINE
NUTRITION
HEALTHY
SPIRIT
CARE

CHAPTER FOUR

Tell me what you eat, and I'll tell you what you are.

–Brillat Savarin

That statement doesn't really apply to fat. Fat doesn't make you fat. Of course, just like thinking or breathing, this much maligned macronutrient can be abused. But that's true of carbs and protein, too. Besides, fat consumption is usually self regulated in the healthy body. Eating fat actually curbs appetite by triggering the release of the hormone cholecystokinin, which causes fullness. If you consume too much of it at one time, you often feel sick. Indeed, there's an old urban legend claiming that it's impossible to drink one gallon of full-fat milk in one hour and keep it down without throwing up. And while I've never tested this theory, I'd assume any validation is partly due to the fat content in whole milk. The same may be true for skim milk, too. But, if so, I imagine that's probably because fat-free milk tastes like watered-down snow-man piss.

No, when fat's abused, it's usually with the type of fat consumed. Or even the type *invented* as happened back in 1911. Originally developed by a German chemist named Edwin C. Kayser in collaboration with Proctor and Gamble, hydrogenated oil—or trans fat as it's commonly called—got its start under the name *Crisco*. The flagship product of P&G was heavily marketed as a replacement for butter and lard—staples in the American diet during the early part of the Twentieth Century. And with the price of these fats soaring, consumers had a financial incentive to look for alternatives.

Hedging their bets, the folks behind Crisco decided to make some dubious health claims, convincing the American people that their plant-based product was healthier than animal fats. As a result, the sales of Crisco exploded while the use of animal fats saw a marked decrease. This trend would continue over the next sixty years with vegetable oil consumption increasing by approximately 400 percent; during this same time, butter fell out of favor with the average American who went from eating eighteen pounds of butter each year to less than four.

One of the first medical practitioners to question the direction the American Diet was moving was a man by the name of Ancel Keys. As early as 1956, he suspected trans fats were responsible for the dramatic increase in coronary thrombosis over the previous decade. The first recorded case of a heart attack didn't occur until 1912 in the *Journal of the American Medical Association*. Since this was just a year after the practice of hydrogenating vegetable oils became popular, maybe Keys was doing nothing more than being observant. Still, Keys was on to something. And had he stuck with that first hunch, perhaps the health history of America may have been different.

17

Widely known as the Father of the so-called *Lipid Hypothesis* wherein dietary fat—and, specifically, saturated fat—causes heart disease, Keys landed his mug on the cover of a 1961 edition of *Time* magazine. By then, he had discarded his earlier theory and used his *Seven Countries Study* to "prove" that saturated fat raises cholesterol and, therefore, is the cause of heart disease.

Now, let's skip over the obvious fallacy of blaming any *one thing* as "the cause" of heart disease or any other illness. For the time being, let's also set aside any discussion of cholesterol since the folklore behind its demonization will require more than a few pages to dispel (that particular debate is discussed in the next chapter). Let us, instead, look a bit more closely at the *Seven Countries Study* to see if anything could've been easily misconstrued.

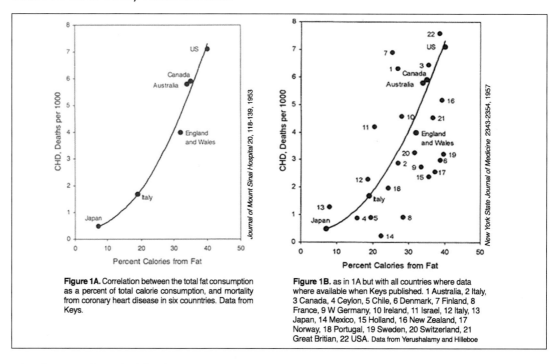

Figure 1A. Correlation between the total fat consumption as a percent of total calorie consumption, and mortality from coronary heart disease in six counntries. Data from Keys.

Figure 1B. as in 1A but with all countries where data where available when Keys published. 1 Australia, 2 Italy, 3 Canada, 4 Ceylon, 5 Chile, 6 Denmark, 7 Finland, 8 France, 9 W Germany, 10 Ireland, 11 Israel, 12 Italy, 13 Japan, 14 Mexico, 15 Holland, 16 New Zealand, 17 Norway, 18 Portugal, 19 Sweden, 20 Switzerland, 21 Great Britian, 22 USA. Data from Yerushalamy and Hilleboe

The first and probably the most glaring problem with the *Seven Countries Study* is that it should have been entitled the *Twenty Two Countries Study*. Keys opted not to include fifteen other countries which may have skewed the results. Among these were countries like France where the proportion of saturated fat in the diet was not coupled with a corresponding increase in coronary heart disease*. Chile was

*This particular oversight would later be explained by the so called "French Paradox", a term coined by French scientist Serge Renaud. Renaud's most celebrated conclusion credited red wine consumption as the secret to French longevity and freedom of disease. Some people, of course, took this information as carte blanche to drink more while others tried to emphasize that moderation was the key. No one, however, seemed to note that Renaud was born in the Bordeaux region of France and the son of a French wine maker...

also excluded. Coronary Heart Disease or CHD (acronyms seem to be much more effective in scaring the population into adhering to any new dietary guidelines or pharmaceutical protocols) was unusually high among the Chileans considering the population's relatively low consumption of fat. Keys also failed to mention that the subjects he used from the island of Crete were in the middle of Lent, during which meat, eggs, and dairy were all off limits. These restrictions would likely have impacted his observation that the Cretan diet was low in saturated fat.

Another potential problem with Keys' work is one inherent to a lot of other studies—association does not equal causation. Epidemiologic research like the *Seven Countries Study* examines the relationship between two (or more) variables. But the more factors at work, the more tenuous any conclusion derived from the results of any particular study. And while researchers today have a number of statistical tools to increase the confidence level of their research, the complexity of the human body existing outside the laboratory environment make causal relationships difficult if not impossible to prove.

Other arguments questioning the validity of the findings from the *Seven Countries Study* could be made. Indeed, many of Keys' own peers noted inconsistencies and flaws in how the research was gathered. But the bandwagon was rolling and Keys' theory was gaining momentum in the scientific community. David Kritchevsky, author of a book entitled *Cholesterol*, published a paper detailing the findings of an experiment he did that involved putting rabbits on high-cholesterol and high-saturated fat diets. The rabbits in the study developed plaques in their arteries, eventually resulting in heart disease and adding more "*evidence*" to the so-called lipid hypothesis. But here's what bugs me: no one ever brought up the fact that rabbits really aren't big meat eaters. Most of the ones I've ever seen are strict vegetarians. Like putting diesel in an unleaded engine, I have to believe that feeding rabbits food better suited for carnivores is just plain Looney Tunes!

What's even crazier is ignoring the critical role saturated fat plays in the human body. Your heart is actually wrapped in it. Indeed, the heart's preferred source of fuel is palmitic acid and stearic acid—both saturated fats. According to one of the premiere experts on the subject of dietary fats and health, Dr. Mary Enig, saturated fat should comprise at least 50% of the total daily fat intake for calcium to be effectively assimilated into the bone structure.

Immune system function is influenced by the presence of saturated fats, too. Butyric acid, a saturated fat found in butter, is the main food source for colonocytes—cells in the lining of the intestines. Studies have shown it to be effective in the treatment of inflammatory bowel diseases like Crohn's, ulcerative colitis, or even colon cancer. Caprylic acid is known for its antiviral properties and has been shown to fight candida. Lauric acid has recently been reported to be beneficial against HIV. From the conclusion of a study entitled *Coconut Oil in Health and Disease: Its and Monolaurin's Potential as a Cure for HIV/AIDS*:

This initial trial confirmed the anecdotal reports that coconut oil does have an anti-viral effect and can beneficially reduce the viral load of HIV patients. The positive anti-viral action was seen not only with the monoglyceride of lauric acid but with coconut oil itself. This indicates that coconut oil is metabolized to monoglyceride forms of C-8, C-10, C-12 to which it must owe its anti-pathogenic activity."

Even respiration depends on saturated fat. A report in PubMed states "*a significant correlation between the impairment of biophysical surfactant function and decreased percentages of palmitic acid was noted.*" Simply stated, fatty acid content impacts the lining and, thus, the health and functioning of the lungs.

YEAH, BUT SATURATED FATS RAISE CHOLESTEROL!

Most blanket statements end up covering the truth. And the one above is no exception. Stearic acid is a saturated fat which actually has *no* adverse impact on cholesterol levels. Second only to palmitic acid as the most abundant saturated fat found in nature, stearic acid is found in foods of animal origin as well as other politically incorrect dietary goodies like cocoa. In the liver, stearic acid is converted via a desaturase enzyme to the 18-carbon monounsaturated oleic acid—the same "*heart healthy*" fat found in olive oil. This conversion may explain why stearic acid is actually associated with reduced levels of LDL—the so called "*bad*" cholesterol. Oleic acid is also found in the myelin of nerve fibers and is essential for the proper development of the entire nervous system. Yes, saturated fat is actually good for the brain. Who woulda thunk it?

YEAH, BUT *MOST* SATURATED FATS RAISE CHOLESTEROL!

While I will admit that statement is true, I would ask the reader to consider this one thought:

So what?

In *Holistic Strength Training for Triathlon* I define posture as the position from which movement begins and ends. My point being that if you begin in the wrong place, you often end in the wrong place. Ideology is no different. And if your set of beliefs is developed on the foundation of faulty premises, the ideas you build will most likely reflect that construction.

Modern dietary dogma is all predicated on the idea that cholesterol—a constituent of *every cell* in your body—is somehow the villain. Indeed, most of us have been so brainwashed by pseudoscience that we're more likely to believe what "a new study finds" than what millions of years of evolution should make abundantly clear.

Cholesterol is not the enemy.

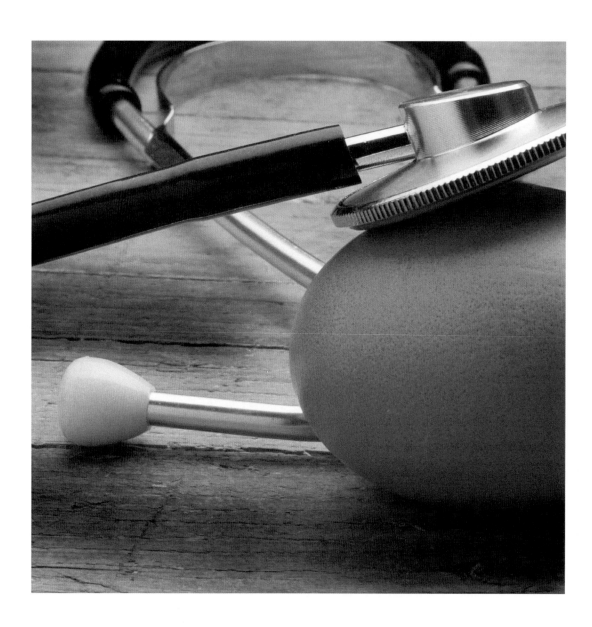

CHAPTER FIVE

Patients should be advised to report promptly any unexplained and/or persistent muscle pain, tenderness, or weakness.

*–Warning Insert for a popular
Statin Drug*

What is the heart?

It's a muscle. And the fine-print disclaimer above is included in the packaging of cholesterol-lowering drugs for a couple of reasons. The first and most obvious is that we are a litigious society, so drug manufacturers must cover their asses. The second one, however, may surprise you. Cholesterol helps heal the body.

Cholesterol is so critical to health that your body readily produces it—making approximately a dozen eggs worth of cholesterol each day. In fact, only about 15% of cholesterol comes from the diet. The remainder is made from acetyl Coenzyme A in the liver and, to some extent, by other cells of the body. Yet, for a dynamic organism constantly working and turning over cells (that would be us), even *this* amount is not sufficient. So the body does something that's rather progressive for a species which is millions of years old: it goes green.

The body is extremely environmentally conscious when it comes to your biological terrain. It recycles key substances whenever and wherever it can. In the case of cholesterol, HDL transports this vital resource back to the liver so it can be used again. Thus, it's become widely known as the "*good*" cholesterol. Of course, mainstream dogma has drowned a lot of victims in misinformation. There really is no such thing as "*good*" cholesterol. Likewise, the only reason cholesterol should be considered "*bad*" is if it somehow gets wasted, steals the keys to your car, and then totals it when trying to outrun the cops.

Cholesterol is just cholesterol.

To get to and from the various tissues in the body, cholesterol needs to have a chaperone of sorts. Not because you can't trust it or it's up to no good. It's simply because oil and water don't mix very well. Specifically, cholesterol is attached to different types of lipoproteins which all have various compositions. Categorized according to the ratio of lipids to protein—the higher the fat, the lower the density—the types of lipoproteins are listed below:

- HDL (high-density lipoprotein)
- LDL (low-density lipoprotein)
- IDL (intermediate-density lipoproteins)
- VLDL (very low-density lipoproteins)
- Chylomicrons (the lowest density lipoprotein)

Early into my indoctrination of politically correct nutrition, I translated the "*H*" in HDL as healthy to help remind me who the good guy was. I also believed that every good guy had to have a bad guy. And while I had been convinced that role was played by LDL, I wasn't all that familiar with the other three *lipoproteins* (or, indeed, the term "lipoprotein"—otherwise I might have been able to figure out what the final "*L*" stood for....). But, looking at the bullet points above, it's not too far fetched to assume that:

- HDL = Healthy
- LDL = Causes Atherosclerosis
- IDL = Related To The Ebola Virus
- VLDL = Very Likely Death Will Occur
- Chylomicrons = Will Explode Your Face Off If Consumed

So why haven't most of us even heard of Chylomicrons? Ignorance may be bliss; but if there's some highly combustible substance in the food we're eating, I wanna know about it! Eventually I started poking around and asking questions. Then you know what I discovered? Those deadly chylomicrons contain hardly any cholesterol! Not even double digits! So that's probably why they're largely ignored. VLDL doesn't matter either, because it's only about 10-15% cholesterol. And IDL—the middle child of the five lipoproteins—has a proportion of cholesterol which is less than impressive. Thus, it really doesn't warrant a lot of attention from doctors (besides, it's not easily measured in a fasting blood test). LDL levels are what the medical community wants to keep in check. After all, even though almost 50% of all patients suffering from heart disease have normal levels of this lipoprotein, LDL is almost *half* cholesterol! And it's *all* about cholesterol:

> *Cholesterol is the most highly decorated small molecule in biology. Thirteen Nobel Prizes have been awarded to scientists who devoted major parts of their careers to cholesterol. Ever since it was isolated from gallstones in 1784, cholesterol has exerted an almost hypnotic fascination for scientists from the most diverse areas of science and medicine....*
> —Michael Brown and Joseph Goldstein from *Nobel Lectures* (1985)

Okay, so let's look at cholesterol then. But this time let's do it from a non-traditional perspective—one which considers the merits of cholesterol and its role, if any, in the maintenance of a healthy human body.

In fact, cholesterol is essential for the health of *any* animal, human or not. Unlike plants which have a cell wall comprised of cellulose, the structural integrity of our cellular membranes relies on an adequate supply of cholesterol. See, one of the most interesting characteristics of cholesterol is it has amphipathic properties. In laymen's terms, this means it contains both hydrophobic and hydrophilic regions. In laymen's *laymen's* terms, this means cholesterol has a part that is "water-fearing" (which makes up the majority of the cholesterol molecule) and not soluble in water; and it also has another part that is "water-loving" and, therefore, water-soluble. This unique yet absolutely critical dichotomy allows the cell membrane to be more resistant to pathogens that could harm the cell, while also being open to vital nutrients involved in cellular functioning.

Cholesterol is also an essential element in the production of bile—another amphipathic substance made by the liver which helps to disperse fat molecules, making them more susceptible to the effect of the pancreatic enzyme lipase. Because let's face it: what good is fat if you can't digest it? And it's digestion which allows the fat-soluble vitamins A, D, E, and K to work their health magic on the human organism.

Speaking of vitamins, D_3 is synthesized by the action of sunlight (UV-B rays) on a precursor to cholesterol called 7-dehydrocholesterol. Though classified as a vitamin, D_3—or cholecalciferol (as opposed to the form found in plant foods, D_2 or ergocalciferol)—actually works much like a hormone and has a myriad of health benefits, which will be explored in a later chapter.

Additionally, dehydroepiandrosterone (DHEA), progesterone, testosterone—indeed, *all* of the body's steroidal hormones use cholesterol as their structural basis. Even cortisol, with its potent anti-inflammatory properties, requires cholesterol as a building block. A glucocorticoid, cortisol has gained infamy as the notorious "stress" hormone. But, trust me—you'd be a lot more stressed if your body couldn't produce it.

A growing body of research suggests that cholesterol may be the ultimate anti-oxidant, too (http://www.ncbi.nlm.nih.gov/pubmed/1937129). When levels are sufficient, cholesterol prevents arachidonic acid—an omega 6 fatty acid—from converting into pro-inflammatory mediators such as thromboxane (as in thrombosis) or leukotriene. One study noted:

> *Cholesterol presents some important characteristics generally ascribed to an antioxidant molecule: its presence in liposomes increases the vesicle resistance to oxidation and its oxidized forms are stable as they are unable to stimulate further propagation of peroxidation reactions. Moreover, the protective effect of cholesterol in liposomes is comparable to that of vitamin E, suggesting that cholesterol possibly acts by intercepting the peroxyl radicals formed during lipid peroxidation.*

One study! What the hell good is one study? There's a load of research out there which says the exact opposite. And besides—when's the last time you saw an advertisement for cholesterol-*raising* medication?

I can't really answer that last question as I don't really watch a lot of TV (having no cable...and a life). But to your point about all the research, I agree that what's out there is a *load*. And while your *"studies"* often cite entities with a financial agenda, my list of references includes a keen understanding of biochemistry and solid common sense. Yet if that's not enough to satisfy your analytical side, perhaps this study's conclusion will:

Lancet. 2001 Aug 4;358(9279):351-5.
Cholesterol and all-cause mortality in elderly people from the Honolulu Heart Program: a cohort study.
The association between reduction of cholesterol concentrations and deaths not related to illness warrants further investigation. Additionally, the failure of cholesterol lowering to affect overall survival justifies a more cautious appraisal of the probable benefits of reducing cholesterol concentrations in the general population.

Or maybe this one will:

Epidemiology. 1997 Mar;8(2):137-43.
Decline in serum total cholesterol and the risk of death from cancer.
The group with the highest decline in cholesterol displayed an excess risk for most cancer sites. These associations were more pronounced in subjects whose weight remained stable or decreased over time than in those who gained weight.

Or this one:

BMJ. 1996 Sep 14;313(7058):649-51.
Serum cholesterol concentration and death from suicide in men: Paris prospective study I.
Both low serum cholesterol concentration and declining cholesterol concentration were associated with increased risk of death from suicide in men.

This one might:

J Am Coll Cardiol. 2003 Dec 3;42(11):1933-40.
The relationship between cholesterol and survival in patients with chronic heart failure.
In patients with CHF, lower serum total cholesterol is independently associated with a worse prognosis.

Or how about this one:

Annals of Internal Medicine March 15, 1998 vol. 128 no. 6 478-487
Cholesterol and Violence: Is There a Connection?

A significant association between low or lowered cholesterol levels and violence is found across many types of studies. Data on this association conform to Hill's criteria for a causal association. Concerns about increased risk for violent outcomes should figure in risk–benefit analyses for cholesterol screening and treatment.

And here's another one if you need:

Scand J Prim Health Care. 2010 Jun;28(2):121-7.
Serum total cholesterol levels and all-cause mortality in a home-dwelling elderly population: a six-year follow-up.
Participants with low serum total cholesterol seem to have a lower survival rate than participants with an elevated cholesterol level, irrespective of concomitant diseases or health status.

I've amassed quite the collection of scientific studies and could show you *pages* if you wanted, but where's that going to get us—nowhere but another impasse. You've got your proof. I've got mine. And like the very arteries we're all worried about, our ability to reason has gotten so clogged up we cannot seem to get unstuck. We're so afraid that there could be more to the story we've been told, that to even entertain another point of view is incredibly dangerous. It's like throwing a clot. And when a belief this big gets dislodged from what we've convinced ourselves we know, our ideology suffers a massive stroke and can never make a complete recovery.

But that's good.

Sometimes it's necessary for something to die before something new can be born. Ideas can be reincarnated into enlightenment. But that evolution can only begin with an open mind—one which allows in thoughts that challenge us; stress our belief system enough to stimulate adaptation.

My transformation began back in college as an aspiring bike racer looking for an edge. The prevailing thought among the endurance community at the time was high carb/low fat. And I was the poster child for that dietary dogma. In one of my classes, we analyzed the macro nutrient profile of my typical daily food intake and found it was incredibly lopsided:

Carbohydrate: **87**%
Protein: **7%**
Fat: **6%**

Now, the testing grounds for that nutritional strategy happened to be the local USCF race scene. While I won't say it was failing miserably, I will admit that I wasn't happy with the results. The analogy I was living far too often—getting chewed up and spat out the back of the pack—eventually got me to question my diet. So I started tweaking what I was putting into my body. Pasta was traded for protein. Skim was replaced with whole. And as the proportion of carbohydrate in my diet decreased, my performance increased exponentially.

My results that season were good enough to earn me an invite to the Olympic Training Center in Colorado. Unfortunately, they weren't good enough to get my coaches to challenge the status quo. Walking into the cafeteria of the OTC, I was bombarded by cereals and grains and pastas galore. The only things more emaciated than the food selection were the athletes themselves. Still, all the cyclists were incredibly strong. And the coaches were adamant their nutritional protocol worked. Ignoring my own instincts, I got in line fast so I wouldn't get dropped.

But that's exactly what happened when I went to Belgium that summer. I would say I was hanging on for dear life across the cobbles of Flanders. Yet the truth is I was suffering too much. The racing was so hard and intense I couldn't seem to keep my tongue off my front wheel, and life is less than endearing with the taste of rubber in your mouth. After the first couple of weeks, I simply wasn't recovering. I went from barely squeezing in to the money to getting shelled out the back like a rotten oyster.

Then one day we raced twice—a road race in the morning followed by a time trial that afternoon. As usual, I sucked in the first event and went to the hotel's dining hall to tap off my depleted glycogen stores. Other racers from various countries were there, and I looked around for any I knew or who might speak English. As I scanned the room, I noticed what the majority of riders had on their plates and almost gagged. Steaks—most of them rather rare—sat atop beds of rice being dyed pink as the cyclists cut into their meat. They devoured their food with two hands and rarely paused to look up, eating as fast as they raced. Their elbows were out like they were protecting their place in the peloton. Not that I was a threat to any of their meals. My coaches had driven a nutritional doctrine so deep inside of me that I was convinced I was going to hammer these gluttonous carnivores in the time trial later that day.

Yet once again I ended up being the nail.

A few more poundings like that and the coffin lid to my cycling dreams was securely in place. I began to wonder what I was even doing over in Europe. What was I spending all this time and energy for? I missed my girlfriend. I missed going to the movies. I became skeptical of everything I'd sacrificed over the past couple of years until I realized what I *really* needed to question.

Convention.

It was high time I put high carb to rest. It wasn't working for me. If I could put it out of its misery, perhaps I could end mine. And if it didn't work out, at least I'd move so far in one direction that I'd realize I was going the wrong way.

That was one of the best moves I've ever made. Not only did my body respond, but my thought process changed as well. On a "new" diet, my cycling results encouraged me that I could make a living racing bikes, and I turned pro. And while that career was short lived, I learned to embrace these transformations of thought on every level of my life. Now when I find ideas that are well past their expiration date, I do the only thing that's truly healthy for me—I throw them out. And I hope I've convinced you to do the same.*

*Apparently some long set beliefs are expiring as I write this. A friend/client of mine posted the following on my Facebook wall: "Andrew Johnston, they finally caught up to you." http://www. forbes.com/.../new-us-guidelines-will-lift-limits.../ If you'll follow the link, it takes you to an article about the 2015 Dietary Guidelines for America in which they reveal the long standing limitations on daily cholesterol intake are being removed. Specifically, the report states "Cholesterol is not considered a nutrient of concern for overconsumption." Well, I'll be! I don't know if I'd say they actually caught up with me but I am impressed. Next thing they'll figure out is that the world isn't flat...

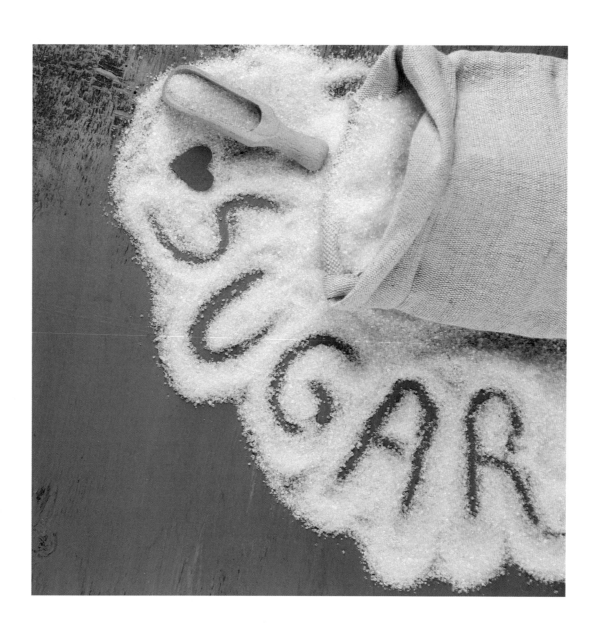

Pour some sugar on me, ooh, in the name of love
Pour some sugar on me, c'mon fire me up
Pour your sugar on me, I can't get enough
I'm hot, sticky sweet from my head to my feet, yeah

—Def Leppard

I don't think anyone in the band Def Leppard was an M.D. As far as I know, none of them even graduated from high school. Still, they were on to something when they wrote *Pour Some Sugar on Me* back in the late 1980's. Think about it. If you're ever in an accident and taken to the emergency room, one of the first things the doctors will do to stabilize you is hook you up to a bag of sugar. Your body loves it. It fires up cellular function. And you cannot get enough of it.

That's right—in addition to being sticky sweet, sugar is addictive. Just like oxygen is addictive. And if you don't get the right amount of either, you die. In the case of sugar, however, quality seems to trump quantity. Or at least that's what's commonly believed. The debate of processed vs. unprocessed or refined vs. unrefined or added vs. naturally occurring—there are as many opinions as there are..., well, grains of sugar. So let's consider some common sources of sugar in the typical diet and how they measure up on the Glycemic Index.

As you may know, the Glycemic Index is a system which ranks various carbohydrates and their impact on blood sugar (i.e., blood glucose). The higher the number, the greater the rise in a person's blood sugar. The concept was developed by David Jenkins, a professor at the University of Toronto who, along with several of his colleagues, authored a study entitled *Glycemic index of foods: a physiological basis for carbohydrate exchange.*

- Glucose   **96**
- French Fries   **95**
- Potato Chips   **90**
- Bread, Gluten Free   **90**
- Rice, Instant   **90**
- Hamburger Buns   **85**
- Potato, Russet   **77**
- Bagel, White   **72**
- Wheat Bread, Wonder   **71**
- Millet   **71**
- White Rice   **70**
- Melba Toast   **70**
- Wheat Bread, Wholemeal   **69**
- Corn Meal   **69**

- Wheat Bread, High Fiber   68
- Taco Shells   68
- Barley Flour Bread   67
- Sucrose (Glucose and Fructose)   64
- High Fructose Corn Syrup   62
- Honey   58
- Orange Juice   52
- Grapefruit Juice   48
- Lactose   46
- Pineapple Juice   46
- Apple   35
- Milk, Whole   30
- Fructose   22

While Dr. Jenkins included 62 different foods in his research, I have opted for an abbreviated list in order to make a point without sacrificing either pages or reader attention. Here's the list again, this time color coded. I've put a key at the bottom to explain why certain colors were used to differentiate the foods listed.

- **Glucose**   96
- French Fries   95
- Potato Chips   90
- Bread, Gluten Free   90
- Rice, Instant   90
- Hamburger Buns   85
- Potato, Russet   77
- Bagel, White   72
- Wheat Bread, Wonder   71
- Millet   71
- White Rice   70
- Melba Toast   70
- Wheat Bread, Wholemeal   69
- Corn Meal   69
- Wheat Bread, High Fiber   68
- Taco Shells   68
- Barley Flour Bread   67
- Sucrose (Glucose and Fructose)   64
- High Fructose Corn Syrup   62
- Honey   58
- Orange Juice   52
- Grapefruit Juice   48
- Lactose   46
- Pineapple Juice   46
- Apple   35
- Milk, Whole   30
- **Fructose**   22

Key:
Bold—monosaccharide (simple sugar molecule)
Red—polysaccharide (chains of glucose molecules)
Blue—disaccharide (combination of glucose and fructose)

Notice anything interesting now when reading the second version? The **bold** denotes a monosaccharide, and there are two listed—**glucose** right at the top with 96 and **fructose** down at the bottom with 22. Both are simple sugar molecules, yet they have dramatically different effects on a person's blood sugar. Cool, huh?

But here's where I *really* want you to pay attention. Check out the foods in red. These are starches, and they're all made up entirely of glucose molecules. For illustrative purposes, they could all look like this:

96-96-96

The blue foods are all a combination of two sugar molecules or *disaccharides*—in this case a pairing of glucose with fructose. So we could say it looks something like this:

96-22

Now, looking at those numbers, is it at all surprising that the red foods create a higher rise in blood sugar than the foods in blue? After all, if you look closely, one of the foods in blue is sucrose—otherwise known as table sugar to you and me. And look what else snuck in there. The darling of the modern day food manufacturer, high fructose corn syrup is also one of the blues!

> *Okay. I get it. You're saying that small increases in blood sugar are bad and large increases are good, right?*

Well...no. No, I'm not. Stick with me here.

As a cyclist, blood sugar has long been a part of my vernacular. What started as pasta on my dinner plate became cereal in my breakfast bowl and eventually found its way into my jersey pockets in the form of power bars and energy gels. These were the days of carbo loading, remember. A cold war had begun in earnest—food companies targeted the athletic market and raced to see how many grams of carbohydrate could be squeezed into a single serving. These concoctions would test the GI fortitude of most any competitor, and countless endurance athletes were humbled by their intestinal limits while stuck in a pre-race port-a-potty.

That's a crappy way to learn that more is not necessarily healthy (pardon the pun). The truth is a large rise in blood sugar is no better or worse than a small increase. Indeed, in the context of the glycemic index, accurate use of qualifiers like "*good*" or "*bad*" or "*healthy*" vs. "*unhealthy*" is predicated on the particular person eating a particular food. More specifically, the impact a certain food has on blood sugar depends on a person's training status, their nutritional status, and a whole host of other factors which can change literally from moment to moment. So why did I even bring up the glycemic index then?

Because *blood sugar is essential.*

It wasn't until I was introduced to a woman named Dodie Anderson that I began to appreciate the truth of that statement. We met through a fellow CHEK Practitioner and good friend of mine named Dan Hellman who suggested I consult her regarding my nutrition and lifestyle strategy as I prepared for the 2012 Great Floridian Iron Distance Triathlon. Dodie happens to be one of the most knowledgeable people I've ever met on the subject of nutrition. Some might go so far as to call her an expert, but that would be doing her a disservice. I've learned that an expert is someone who knows more and more about less and less until they know absolutely everything about nothing. But Dodie wasn't so blind. Our conversations had no limits as we discussed every possible idea remotely related to health and performance. Yet regardless of where our weekly discussions took us, we would always return to the subject of blood sugar.

There's always a sweet spot in which optimal performance occurs. In the realm of athletics it's often called *"the zone."* The term used when referencing blood sugar doesn't have quite the same flare. It's not dramatic or cool sounding at all, in fact. Actually, it's *"normal."*

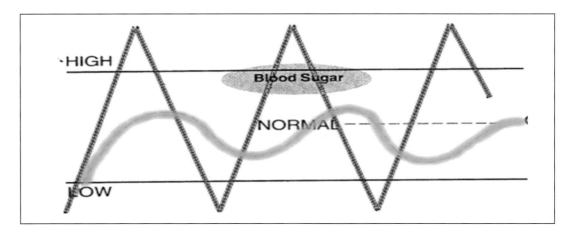

"Normal" blood sugar when in a fasted state is defined 70-100 milligrams per deciliter. It goes up when you eat, of course, but generally no higher than about 135-140mg/dl. Now, that's a fairly small range, so you might think you need to invest in a device you can use to test your blood. But I have a different suggestion. How bout you just listen to your body? It's a bit old school, sure—but it's also a lot less invasive. And it's quite accurate, too, especially when you become proficient at recognizing your body's signals. When blood sugar levels are in the normal rage, you should feel *healthy.* Specifically, you should feel emotionally stable with good energy and clarity of thought. Now, that may be a little too ambiguous for some of you. Or perhaps it's

been so long since you were healthy you can't really remember what it's actually like to feel that way anymore. If that's the case, here's a short list of symptoms so you'll at least know how you *shouldn't* feel:

Wired but tired
Unusual thirst
Polyphagia (pronounced hunger)
Nervous
Jittery
Cravings for fat/protein
Anxious
Sluggish
Sleepy
Lethargic
Irritable
Depressed
Cravings for sugar/carbohydrate/caffeine
Cold

As you'll notice, I color coded the symptoms above to delineate between high and low blood sugar. But there is definitely a lot of crossover between the two, and just about any of the ones listed could fall in either camp. Typically, a person with blood sugar handling problems will present with complaints from both blue *and* red as the body tries desperately to find homeostasis. Constantly bouncing around between low blood sugar and high blood sugar, this rollercoaster doesn't stop until nutrition (and lifestyle) is properly addressed.*

- Carbohydrate raises blood sugar
- Protein lowers blood sugar
- Fat mediates the response to both carbohydrate and protein

The etiology of high blood sugar could be as simple as an imbalanced macronutrient profile at a meal. However, hyperglycemia can have its roots in a host of other factors, as well—many of them quite complex and deserving of their own discussion. Either way, one condition begets the other in a body always seeking homeostasis. So for the sake of simplicity, I will focus the remainder of this chapter on the subject of low blood sugar.

A quick story to illustrate my point. One of my son's friends was constantly bringing home "red lights" from school, indicative of behavior which was unacceptable. In contrast, my son was consistently bringing home "green lights". Yet, I assure you—he's no angel. He's just a normal seven year old boy who can easily push my, admittedly, all too readily accessible buttons. So when the kid's mother became a client of mine, I felt comfortable suggesting dietary changes I thought might help. It was obvious to me my son's friend was having blood sugar handling problems due to a lack of protein and fat both at breakfast and with other meals. She followed my advice, got her doctor to write a note prescribing her son be allowed a small snack during the school day, and it's been mostly green lights ever since...

As you'll remember from a few pages ago, I used the scenario of a trip to the emergency room to illustrate how important sugar is. Without it, you die. But the body is sharply focused on the present. It will sacrifice long term health for short term survival, doing anything it takes to stay alive. And in the case of low blood sugar, it takes one for the team. Or, if you really want the gory details, it *eats* one for the team.

That's right. When you don't provide the fuel for the body, your body becomes the fuel for you. Quite simply, when blood glucose levels decline, the body is forced to dine on fat and protein—*your* fat and protein. And one thing you need to know about human physiology is that, outside of a meal at your parent's house, there's no such thing as a free lunch. So tapping into your protein containing tissues to supply needed energy (or, *yes*, even your own seemingly unlimited fat stores) comes at a cost.

The Price of Protein

Gluconeogenesis is the process of making new (*neo*) sugar from non-carbohydrate sources. A protective action taken to ensure that ATP synthesis can continue, it usually refers to the catabolism of protein but, technically, it includes the breakdown of lipids as well. Though not necessarily your body's first choice of fuel when glucose supplies are limited, I've opted to discuss the catabolism of proteins before I talk about the breakdown of fats (mainly as it'll help me segue into the next chapter). Besides, fat loss is a common goal of individuals engaged in dieting or exercise. So I think the sticker shock of using protein for fuel may prove a bit more dramatic.

When forced to scavenge protein tissues for fuel, the ideal source for your body to find it is in the muscles. You may disagree, of course. Maybe you like big butts and you cannot lie.* But here's something you cannot deny: the body is nothing if not practical. It can live without movement (not *well*, perhaps—but that's another matter). What it doesn't do so great without is something like a liver or a heart. In fact, *all* the organs take higher priority over the muscles of the body. I guess that's another example of how function trumps aesthetics. So the first thing to go is your muscle followed closely by your metabolism:

> *"If it [carbohydrate] is not in the diet, then body protein catabolism will be accelerated for gluconeogenesis. In some individuals, sufficient protein destruction will result to provide glucose for synthesis of substantial quantities of new body fat."*
> —Constance Martin, PhD

But the reason your basal metabolic rate (BMR) takes a hit is not exactly what you might expect. While a pound of muscle burns about three times the number of calories at rest each day as the same amount of fat, losing that contribution to your

Anytime you have a book which references Sir-Mix-a-Lot, you know you're reading quality material.

calorie cap isn't as detrimental to your waistline as you might believe. Fat only adds about two calories per pound per day to your BMR. So if you do the math:

$$3 \times 2 = 6$$

you'll see that muscle really has nothing to brag about. Six calories per pound per day—big whoop!

As you learned in the section on Thoughts of *Spot On*, the brain consumes a lot of energy—accounting for as much as 20% of a person's BMR. The heart, the liver, and the kidneys are right up there, too. *These are where the fires of your metabolism are really stoked.* Muscle's contribution is rather humble in comparison. Yet, as Albert Einstein reportedly said, "*...not everything that counts can be counted.*"

Tryptophan* is one of the major amino acids released when muscle tissue is broken down during gluconeogenesis. Along with cysteine and methionine—two other amino acids liberated during the catabolism of muscle tissue—tryptophan inhibits thyroid peroxidase (TPO). And this is where the *true* price of using protein for fuel becomes increasingly clear. TPO is an enzyme which helps produce thyroid hormone. The thyroid, of course, is the master of metabolism. Metabolism is energy production. And you already know what happens when energy production decreases.

When Energy Production goes down, Adrenaline goes up.
When Adrenaline goes up, Intestinal Circulation (of glucose and O_2) goes down.
When Intestinal Circulation goes down, Endotoxin Production goes up.
When Endotoxin Production goes up, Liver Function goes down.
When Liver Function goes down, Toxic Load goes up.
When Toxic Load goes up, Energy Production goes down.

And you thought grass-fed beef was expensive!

The only reason the body does *anything* is it wants to survive. In this case, the body is trying to spare its own tissues which are being "eaten" to maintain sufficient levels of glucose to keep your biological system functioning. The amino acids released when the main dish you're serving is your body's own protein are a signal that the thyroid needs to be down regulated. So your body turns its "idle" down, giving you a greater chance of making it to the next fill up before completely running out of gas.

---

*Another hidden cost of using the body's muscles to make glucose: tryptophan is metabolized in the body via two different pathways. One converts it to niacin (Vitamin B3). However, if calcium intake is inadequate, the other conversion path results in the production of serotonin and melatonin. What's wrong with that? If you'll hold that thought for a moment, we'll return to it later. For now, suffice it to say that both of these hormone have a darker side—one requiring its own chapter.

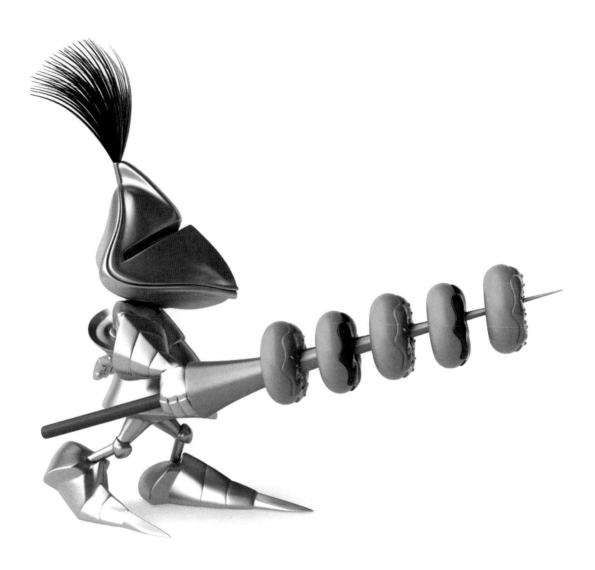

It's an uncommonly dangerous thing to be left without any padding against the shafts of disease.

—George Eliot

The day when you see Jenny Craig in a soup line or *24hr Fitness* closing its doors is probably a long way away. Fat loss is big business. And with two-thirds of the world's population overweight or obese, folks in the industry are enjoying some serious job security. Though it's not just the calorie conscious driving this commerce. Even the athletic community weighs in on the subject of fat, and the general consensus is *the leaner the better*. Fat needs to be annihilated. It should be burned or blasted away! Athletes need to be shredded. Models and actors have to be cut. The terminology used in the war on fat is one which conjures up images of violence, and lipolysis is the weapon everyone's trying to master.

Just make sure you don't end up bringing a knife to a gun fight.

The *real* fight in this case is one for survival. When blood sugar drops—whether from increased demand or insufficient supply—stored fat is used to keep your biological system running. Specifically, triglycerides are broken down into glycerol and three fatty acids molecules. What happens next is where things get interesting.

DEFCON FIVE

Glycerol is converted to glyceraldehyde phosphate to enter what's called the Krebs Cycle. Also known as the Citric Acid Cycle (Citric Acid because citric acid is the first substrate of this cycle; and Krebs because the man who discovered it was named Hans Krebs—I'll stick with Krebs cycle as it's easier to type), the Krebs Cycle is a chemical process which results in the production of ATP. However, glyceraldehyde is only equal to half a glucose molecule ($C_3H_6O_3$), so the net ATP resulting from its oxidation is approximately half that of glucose (18-19 ATP for glycerol vs. 36-38 for glucose). That's the first strike against lipolysis—less energy production. And in case you don't remember, here's the Seesaw of Sickness* again:

Maybe we should put these lines to music so we can remember it better—something like Helter Skelter, perhaps...

When Energy Production goes down, Adrenaline goes up.
When Adrenaline goes up, Intestinal Circulation (of glucose and O_2) goes down.
When Intestinal Circulation goes down, Endotoxin Production goes up.
When Endotoxin Production goes up, Liver Function goes down.
When Liver Function goes down, Toxic Load goes up.
When Toxic Load goes up, Energy Production goes down.

DEFCON FOUR

The three fatty acids are eventually converted (*"beta oxidized"* if you wanna get technical) into two-carbon acetic acid molecules. Each of these fragments then combines with coenzyme A to form acetyl CoA which is picked up by oxaloacetic acid, allowing it entry into the Krebs Cycle.

But (and you should have known there was a *"but"* coming) oxaloacetic acid is converted to glucose during carbohydrate deficit. After all, *something's* gotta fuel the brain. And while fatty acids may be the preferred source of fuel for the heart, the liver, and even *resting* skeletal muscle, the brain is kind of a carbo-holic. It's truly addicted to sugar. It needs its glucose, man! Thus, since acetyl CoA's chaperone into the Krebs Cycle is being used to give the brain its fix, fat oxidation remains incomplete. Ruh-oh!

While all this may sound super complicated, here's an easy way to use your own experience to grasp this concept better than I or any textbook could ever hope to teach it. Simply sign up for a marathon or a century bike ride; then try to go the distance on no food. The wall you hit will be the perfect teacher, and you'll recognize it by how hard it is (some of the best-learned lessons in life often are). Yet even though you may think this mother of all bonks is just due to a lack of calories, that's really your glucose-deprived brain impairing your cognitive abilities. You know even the leanest of athletes has enough calories stored as fat to run back-to-back marathons. Heck, many of us have enough adipose tissue to fuel our own version of the Tour de France. Yet that fat can't do anything for you if you can't access it. Fat burns in a carbohydrate flame.* Science says so. And so does your body.

DEFCON THREE

So what happens to all that left over acetyl CoA if it can't be used in the Krebs Cycle? I'm glad I wrote you asked that. Well, through a process called ketogenesis, the liver converts the excess acetyl CoA molecules into ketone bodies. These ketone bodies—*acetoacetic acid, beta-hydroxybutyric acid,* and *acetone*—are then released into the blood and used as a glucose substitute by extra-hepatic tissues, specifically the brain. This happens every time you're in a fasted state—like during sleep or even

Another reason you "hit the wall" is due to the fact that sugar is the only molecule that can be broken down without oxygen. The more your glucose reserves became depleted, the more reliant you became on the oxidative (aerobic) system which predominates at lower intensities— forcing you to slow down.

long periods between meals—so ketosis is not a condition which needs to be avoided. Indeed, unless you're tied to an I.V. twenty-four seven, you probably switch back and forth between a state of glycolysis (sugar splitting) and a state of ketosis as part of your normal biological rhythm.

The problem begins when ketosis is your default state. See, since most of the ketone bodies are acids, excessive production can overburden the systems that maintain acid/base homeostasis in the body. When this happens, blood pH can drop to dangerously low levels and coma or even death can result. However, except in extreme cases (i.e., untreated type 1 diabetes), this rarely occurs. So maybe we can decrease our alert status back to DEFCON Four?

Mmmm...not so quick.

Your main issue is how your body buffers these acids, and one of its strategies is to hyperventilate. In an effort to raise pH, the body increases its breathing rate so that more CO_2 is expelled. But, unfortunately, this causes oxygen delivery to be reduced. Then blood vessels constrict. And very quickly the Seesaw of Sickness is once again set in motion.*

DEFCON TWO

As luck would have it (though I'll credit my writing skills in this case), the importance of CO_2 is a nice segue to DEFCON Two. Consider the below illustrations comparing two fatty acids and one carbohydrate:

Additionally, the Autonomic Nervous System gets out of balance as overstimulation of the Sympathetic Nervous System inhibits the activity of the Parasympathetic Nervous System (see p. 231-237 in Holistic Strength Training for Triathlon).

Sucrose

Notice how few molecules of oxygen those fatty acids have? This means that burning fat for fuel produces less CO_2 than burning carbohydrate because fatty acids are oxygen poor. Less production coupled with excessive loss means the body is working in a serious CO_2 deficit. If you haven't already figured it out, you can refresh your memory of the importance of CO_2 by referring to the Respiration section of *Spot On*. But to save you time, I'll give you the CliffsNotes version—*as more CO_2 is lost, health becomes increasingly difficult to find.*

DEFCON ONE

Chapter Six was where I had intended to discuss the importance of blood sugar. Of course, I've explored a lot of rabbit holes during the past several pages, so I can understand if I lost any of my readers since we began. The truth is you really don't have to dig too far before you realize that everything is connected. If I pull on your toes, your eyelashes wiggle. So, too, the relationships between all the systems of the body—from the endocrine system to the respiratory system—are intimately intertwined. Thus, writing about blood sugar can cause someone as tangentially inclined as myself to go off in approximately a million different directions at once. But if you'll stick with me, I'll bring it all back together soon (or later...).

Right now I'd like to address what may be the most important reason lipolysis is a faulty strategy when it comes to survival. And in an effort to keep it simple, I'll condense the problem down to just one word: PUFA.

Okay, so, yes—technically, PUFA is an acronym and not specifically a word. But condensing the problem down to "*just four letters*" didn't sound as powerful. So I hope you'll let me slide on that one.

Standing for Polyunsaturated Fatty Acids, PUFAs have grown increasingly common in the Standard American Diet. What began as (misguided) health advice from Ancel Keys soon became the rallying cry of the United State's war on obesity and its related diseases. The Dietary Guidelines of the U.S. Department of Agriculture were put into place

at a time of rising concern about the health of the American population. Poor diet and physical inactivity are the most important factors contributing to an epidemic of overweight and obesity affecting men, women, and children in all segments of our society. Poor diet...[is also] linked to major causes of illness and death. To correct these problems, many Americans must make significant changes in their eating habits....

Their recommendations were clear:

To reduce the intake of saturated fatty acids, many Americans should limit their consumption of the major sources that are high in saturated fatty acids and replace them with foods that are rich in monounsaturated and polyunsaturated fatty acids. For example, when preparing foods at home, solid fats (e.g., butter and lard) can be replaced with vegetable oils that are rich in monounsaturated and polyunsaturated fatty acids

And look what happened:

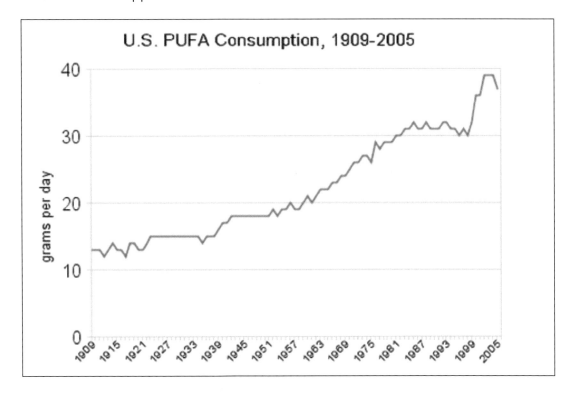

PUFA consumption exploded! And so did our waistlines, with more than two-thirds of Americans now considered overweight or obese. Of course, we were simply doing what our benevolent government told us to do. So perhaps I should have condensed the problem down to a different acronym: USDA. But I'm really not trying to throw any government entity under the bus (they're doing a fine job of that entirely on their own). Besides, that's a subject well beyond the scope of this book. I've always had more of a taste for nutrition than politics. So, if you don't mind, let's keep our focus on the problem with PUFAs.

As discussed earlier, glucose is the fuel of choice for the brain. Fatty acids are unable to pass the blood-brain barrier. Additionally, thiolase—the enzyme responsible for cleaving acetyl CoA off the rest of the fatty acid at the end of beta oxidation—is found in extremely limited quantities in the neurons of the brain; thus, levels of acetyl CoA are not sufficient to run the Krebs Cycle. So for the brain, it's essentially sugar or bust. Red blood cells, lacking any mitochondria, also cannot function without glucose. And various other parts of the body use glucose exclusively, too (i.e., the retina).

The issue with PUFAs is they have a strong influence on the body's ability to use glucose for fuel. By "*strong influence,*" I mean they don't let it happen. Specifically, PUFAs have been shown to block the action of pyruvate dehydrogenase,* an enzyme involved in the aerobic metabolism of sugar. Interfering with *any* of the glycolytic steps is actually just a basic survival strategy long ago encoded into our biochemistry. Termed glucose sparing, this essential process helped keep us alive during periods of starvation—a possible and perhaps even probable condition humans encountered at various times in our evolutionary history. If critical bodily functions are dependent on a supply of glucose, having a back up plan when quantities are limited is probably a smart idea.

These days, of course, a famished state is often one that is self-induced. Strict diets, overzealous exercise regimens, or even simply being to busy to eat can all decrease blood sugar and trigger heightened levels of alarm in the body. And while lipolysis may have helped our ancestors to survive during times of scarcity, the overwhelming percentage of PUFAs in today's diet makes this protective mechanism more one of mutually assured destruction when used by modern man.

Was that last statement supplied with too generous a dose of hyperbole? I *was* a Creative Writing major, so that observation might not be entirely inaccurate. However, in this case at least, I am really not exaggerating. Indeed, the somewhat strained war analogy I've been using during the course of this chapter is quite appropriate when one considers how Ray Peat views polyunsaturated fatty acids. His list of the worst metabolic offenders can be seen below:

1. **PUFAs**
2. **Radiation**
3. **Darkness**
4. **Over Exercising**
5. **Lack of Digestible Fuel (e.g., glucose/protein)**

Basically, based off Dr. Peat's expert opinion, you've got a better chance of surviving a nuclear holocaust with your health intact than consuming a lot of PUFAs.

You may think I'm overstating the danger. Or maybe it's time someone revoked my

---

Interestingly, saturated fats actually help to activate this crucial enzyme.

poetic license. But the fact is PUFAs have a host of deleterious effects we haven't even covered yet. And by now you're probably asking yourself how bad these little fatty acids could be.

Well, let me channel my inner Elizabeth Barrett Browning and say, *"let me count the ways..."*

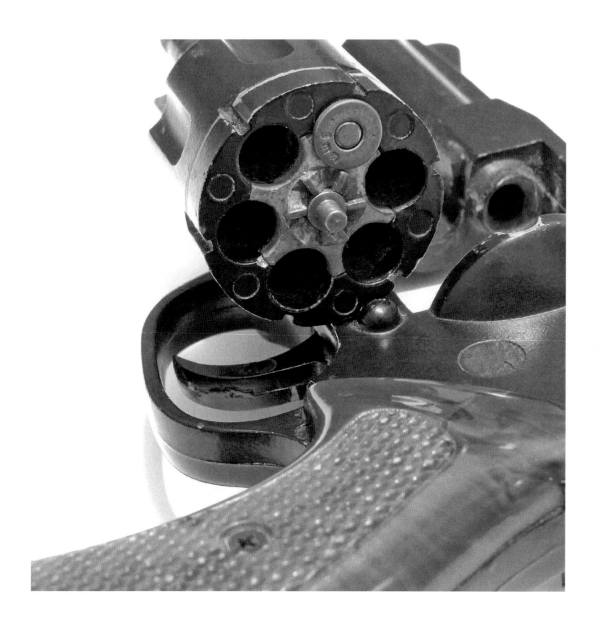

CHAPTER SEVEN

Everyone should have the privilege of playing Russian roulette if it is desired, but it is only fair to have the warning that with the use of polyunsaturated fats the gun probably contains live ammunition.

—Broda Barnes

Stop picking on PUFAs!

Those of my readers familiar with the Randle Cycle* may contend that *all* types of dietary fat interfere with the oxidation of carbohydrate, so why am I singling out polyunsaturated fatty acids? The answer to that question begins by referencing the graph from the last chapter. As PUFAs replaced saturated fat in our diet, our bodies' fat stores began to reflect that change. Thus, anytime lipolysis occurred, the fats which we utilized were these very same PUFAs.

The source of fat used, however, is influenced by more than just availability. PUFAs are more water-soluble than either monounsaturated or saturated fat. Thus, they are released more readily into the aqueous environment of the bloodstream when compared to either of these types of fats. Additionally, with more carbon links left unsaturated, PUFAs have greater exposure to both hormone sensitive lipase (HSL) and lipoprotein lipase (LPL)—lipolytic enzymes which trigger the mobilization of triglycerides from various storage sites in the body. So when lipolysis is initiated, PUFAs are typically the first in line.

With an endogenous supply now mirroring out exogenous intake, we are literally poisoning ourselves from both ends. And I don't use that term lightly. Yeah, *"poisoning"* is a strong word. But it's probably found less frequently in my vocabulary than it's found in your food, especially if your diet contains any of the following:

canola oil	**nuts/nut butters**
corn oil	**seeds**
cotton seed oil	**sesame oil**
fish oil	**sunflower oil**
flaxseed oil	**vegetable oil**
margarine	

I know what you're thinking. With the exception of margarine, all the above listed items are completely natural. Well, to some extent that's true. However, well before the label of *"natural"* was ever abused by the food manufacturing industry, the term

In short, the Randle cycle holds that the utilization of one nutrient (e.g., fat) inhibits the utilization of another nutrient (e.g., carbohydrate).

was one which didn't necessarily grant the human digestive system cart blanche to what it could be exposed to. Our predecessors discovered this truth over countless generations of trial and error. And while some mistakes were paid for simply with a sour stomach, other times the cost was much higher.

See, there's nothing in Nature which really *wants* to die. Animals typically use fangs or claws or speed to defend themselves. Plants, however, don't share these same types of rudimentary protection. Instead they've developed other methods—some of them quite ingenious—to ensure their survival. For example, cotton plants emit a substance that can attract predatory wasps when damaged by moth larvae. Spinach produces a type of steroid to protect it from nematodes and other parasites by disrupting larval development and increasing insect mortality (maybe that's why Popeye was always able to kick Bluto's ass after downing a can...). There are an infinite number of other examples found in Nature which prove that all life invariably wants to continue. Even the smallest or seemingly non-sentient of living creatures has learned to protect themselves against predators higher up on the food chain. And PUFAs—at least in light of current nutritional guidelines—have become by far the most dangerous of the chemical defenses commonly found in the diet of modern man.

IMMUNOSUPPRESSIVE

When an animal gets sick in the wild, its chances of dying increase exponentially. Thus, an excellent way a plant can ensure its own survival is by suppressing the immune system of whatever may dine on it. After all, dead predators don't really eat a whole lot. And even if the animal is lucky enough to survive, feeling sick typically puts quite a dent on its appetite. Immunosuppression is one of the effects PUFAs have on an organism's biochemistry. And, ironically, it's why many of these oils are touted as being good for us.

Inflammation is one response of a functioning immune system. After a physical trauma or even an attack by a specific pathogen, the injured cells release various chemicals (e.g., histamine) which induce swelling. This helps isolate the damaged area from other parts of the body while at the same time attracting white blood cells called phagocytes to come "*clean up*" the mess.

Inhibit the immune system, and inflammation is reduced. This concept has led to an entire industry of medical and exercise professionals advocating the use of PUFAs as a treatment for inflammatory conditions ranging from arthritis to heart disease to asthma. But could this philosophy be shortsighted? Is it possible we are so focused on treating inflammation that we're losing sight of long term health? Luckily, I'm not the first person to consider that question:

Am J Clin Nutr. 1991 Apr;53(4 Suppl):1064S-1067S.
Dietary fats and cancer.
Experiments on animals have indicated that polyunsaturated vegetable oils promote cancer more effectively than do saturated fats

Lancet. 1994 Oct 29;344(8931):1195-6.
Dietary polyunsaturated fatty acids and composition of human aortic plaques.
These findings imply a direct influence of dietary polyunsaturated fatty acids on aortic plaque formation and suggest that current trends favouring increased intake of polyunsaturated fatty acids should be reconsidered.

Cancer Res. 1998 Aug 1;58(15):3312-9.
Dietary omega-3 polyunsaturated fatty acids promote colon carcinoma metastasis in rat liver.
At 3 weeks after tumor transplantation, the fish oil diet and the safflower oil diet had induced, respectively, 10- and 4-fold more metastases (number) and over 1000- and 500-fold more metastases (size) than were found in the livers of rats on the low-fat diet.... In conclusion, omega-3 and omega-6 PUFAs promote colon cancer metastasis in the liver....

Nutrition. 2004 Feb;20(2):230-4.
Diets rich in saturated and polyunsaturated fatty acids: metabolic shifting and cardiac health.
PUFAs have been recommended as a therapeutic measure in preventive medicine to lower serum cholesterol, but PUFAs increased oxidative stress in the heart by providing cardiac susceptibility to lipoperoxidation and shifting the metabolic pathway for energy production.

Cancer and plaques and lipoperoxidation—Oh my!   Scores and perhaps even hundreds of studies come to the same conclusion, but most are either ignored or purposely misinterpreted to support a specific position. And while the truth may not be as easy to follow as a yellow brick road, the facts are supported in the literature for anybody with half a brain and the courage to look. Indeed, once you do, you'll typically find the researchers behind the curtain of many of the studies are wizards at manipulating data for their own personal agenda. I'll let my man Ray Peat have the last word here:

In declaring EPA and DHA to be safe, the FDA neglected to evaluate their antithyroid, immunosuppressive, lipid peroxidative (Song et al., 2000), light sensitizing, and antimitochondrial effects, their depression of glucose oxidation (Delarue et al., 2003), and their contribution to metastatic cancer (Klieveri, et al., 2000), lipofuscinosis and liver damage, among other problems.

PRO-INFLAMMATORY

The body is always striving for homeostasis. Anytime the human organism is chronically out of balance, health is what suffers. Traditional diets are believed to have provided Omega-3 fats and Omega-6* fats in a ratio of 1:1. But a little over a hundred years ago, sometime shortly after the industrial revolution, that balance began to change. Vegetable oil consumption along with the increased use of cereal grains in the diet of both humans and livestock shifted that ratio in favor of Omega-6 fatty acids; the current estimates show our current ratio in the United States to be 1:15. Some research shows that statistic to be as skewed as 1:25. Whichever calculation you use, one fact cannot be argued: arthritis, heart disease, and many other conditions related to excessive inflammation are now epidemic. In one of the most extensive analyses performed to date, authors of a 2012 research study entitled *Fatty acid composition of membrane bilayers: Importance of diet polyunsaturated fat balance* wrote:

> ...this low diet PUFA balance is of grave concern, with an imbalance between diet n-3 and n-6 PUFA associated with a number of diseases which have become prevalent in today's society, such as dyslipidaemia, hypertension, inflammation, depression, abdominal obesity, type 2 diabetes and cardiovascular disease [[7], [36], [37] and [38]]. In particular, chronic inflammation is known to be the driving force behind many diseases that have increased in recent time, including insulin resistance, obesity, atherosclerosis, cancer and neurodegenerative diseases, such as Alzheimer's disease [39] and [40]. Diet fatty acid composition is known to influence inflammation through changes in cell membrane fatty acid composition, with changes in the substrate availability for pro-inflammatory eicosanoids (from 20:4n-6) and anti-inflammatory resolvins and protectins (from 20:5n-3 and 22:6n-3) [40]. So an imbalance towards too much n-6 PUFA in the modern human diet may result in increased membrane 20:4n-6 levels and thus increased chronic inflammation in many humans.

Now, there's nothing wrong with omega-6—and that's a good thing because they're literally everywhere. So you can't avoid them completely. It's getting too much of them in your diet that you want to avoid. Specifically, it's the omega-6 fatty acid Arachidonic Acid (AA) you want to look out for. In descending order, the foods which supply the majority of this fatty acid in the American diet are:

*Omega-3 fatty acids and Omega-6 fatty acids are both forms of PUFAs. As such, they both have more than one double bond in the carbon chain. It's the location of the first double bond counted from the methyl end (CH3) which determines how a particular PUFA is classified. For example, DHA, or Docosahexaenoic Acid, is a 22-carbon chain fatty acid with the first of its six double bonds found at the third carbon from the omega end; thus, it is referred to as an Omega-3. Linoleic Acid, or LA, is an Omega-6 fatty acid since its first double bond occurs at the sixth carbon from the omega end.

1. Poultry
2. Eggs
3. Red Meat*

Ultimately, however, the majority of your exposure to Arachidonic Acid is derived from Linoleic Acid (LA) which, though a complex series of desaturation and elongation reactions, is converted into AA in the body. Thus, a more prudent approach may simply to be more cognizant of the common sources of LA in the foods we eat.

Now if you have neither the time nor the inclination to figure out where Linoleic Acid is most readily found in your diet, simply take the American Heart Association's recommendations:

- *"Use naturally occurring, unhydrogenated vegetable oils such as canola, safflower, sunflower or olive oil most often."*
- *"Use soft margarine as a substitute for butter...."*
- *"Eat a dietary pattern that emphasizes...whole grains...."*

And do the exact opposite.

Unless, of course, you *want* excessive production of pro-inflammatory eicosanoids prostaglandin E2 (PGE2) and leukotriene B4 (LTB4).** If that's the case, then you will find no better fuel to fan the flames of disease and dysfunction than the guidelines of the AHA (the recommendations of the USDA could probably be considered just as combustible, but those two organizations are more/less one in the same).

The current treatment model for fighting excessive inflammation among most is the use of NSAIDs. Second only to cholesterol lowering drugs (though with the popularity of pharmaceuticals in the United States, this statistic could easily be outdated at the time of this reading), Non-Steroidal Anti-Inflammatories are quick, easy, moderately effective, and have little risk of complication...until you read the fine print. But some forward thinking folks with an interest in health suggested an alternative—supplement with omega 3's. Their reasoning was sound. Consuming large amounts of Omega 3's (typically derived from fish oil or flax seed oil) results in a partial replacement of AA in the cell membrane with both DHA and eicosapentaenoic acid (EPA); this leads to decreased production of the AA-derived mediators which, as you now know, tend to be pro-inflammatory. In addition, because EPA and AA have the same number

Note that pastured/free range animal products contain less AA than conventionally raised counterparts fed with commercial feed. This, of course, is due to the differences in diet between the two. Change the diet, and you change the nutrient content of the animal eating the diet. This concept applies to humans and what we eat, as well.

**NSAIDs "work" by suppressing the formation of inflammatory compounds made from omega-6 fatty acids. By limiting the action of cyclooxygenase (one of the enzymes responsible for converting AA into pro-inflammatory eicosanoids), inflammation is inhibited. This process has a downside, too, of course.*

of carbon atoms, EPA competes for the exact enzymes which metabolize AA. The premise was simple: less fuel=less flame.

Well, those researchers got the *"less flame"* part right...

ANTI-THYROID

Do a search for PUFAs and thyroid, and you'll uncover countless articles which explain that the polyunsaturated fatty acids suppress thyroid function. Unfortunately, you won't see a whole lot out there about *how* or *why* any thyroid inhibition actually occurs. What you will find are anecdotal reports explaining that PUFAs (specifically corn oil and soy oil) were used in the 1940's as an inexpensive way to fatten cattle and other livestock, supposedly by down regulating the thyroid. Today, of course, they're being used by the processed food industry as a cheap way to fatten people. But I digress...If you dig deep enough, you may even discover some studies like the one entitled *Inhibition of triiodothronine's induction of rat liver lipogenic enzymes by dietary fat.* Now, this one's a real page turner! And while the authors don't use terminology readily accessible to the layman, they do conclude that *"...polyunsaturated fats uniquely suppress the gene expression of lipogenic enzymes by functioning as competitive inhibitors of T_3 action, possibly at the nuclear receptor level."*

To dumb that down a bit: PUFAs ain't good if you're a thyroid fan.

And you should be a big thyroid supporter. Sure, most of us consider thyroid function solely in terms of its influence on weight. But it's so much more. This little butterfly-shaped gland found in the front of the lower neck is literally the Master of Metabolism. Much more than thick or thin, metabolism is how each of the more than 100 *trillion* cells in your body is functioning. Indeed, every single biological process is impacted in one way or another by the thyroid. And it's a two way street, too— anything you do at any moment has an effect on your thyroid, including the amount of PUFAs on your plate.

PUFAs block all three proteins—albumin, thyroxine-binding globulin, transthyretin— responsible for carrying thyroxine (T_4) and triiodothyronine (T_3) in the bloodstream. During my research for this book, I learned that markers of thyroid dysfunction are typically found in most chronic diseases. I later found an interesting study on the effects of fatty acid administration on plasma thyroid hormones (okay, so I'm probably not a lot of fun to hang out with, I'll admit). The authors of this particular study make some observations which prove insightful on the interplay between thyroid, health, and PUFAs:

> *"Studies in man...have demonstrated that severe illness is associated with an increase in serum concentrations of free fatty acids...and that they are associated with a reduction in concentrations of serum thyroxine (T_4) and/or triiodothyronine (T_3)."*

When necessary, the body activates the Sympathetic Nervous System (SNS) to prepare for fight or flight. Those two choices—doing battle or running away—both require enormous amounts of energy, much of which can be found in the body's fat stores. Luckily, adipose tissue has a generous supply of sympathetic fibers. Thus, when epinephrine is released by the adrenal medulla in response to stress, this hormone (commonly referred to as adrenalin) stimulates lipolysis to increase circulating levels of fatty acids for use as fuel.

In this scenario, like most others, the body is simply doing what it always does when faced with any type of stressor—trying to adapt. Illness is the stress in this case. So basal metabolic rate is depressed secondary to the release of the anti-thyroid PUFAs into circulation and the caloric cost of keeping the organism alive is therefore lowered. Additionally, PUFAs' inhibition of glucose spares the body's preferred yet limited supply of glycogen so it can access this reserve to fight or flee in the future. That is, if there *is* a future. The body's primary concern is making it through the moment, through right now. Short term survival at all costs—including long term health.

FISH OIL

Everyone knows eating fish is good for you. But for those who don't, the America Heart Association advises to *"try a serving once a week, preferably twice."* The logic is simple, if something is good for you, then more good = better!* In addition, as the former chair of the AHA's Nutrition Committee Dr. Alice Lichtenstein points out, *"whenever you eat fish, you are cutting something else from your diet, particularly other protein sources that may be less healthy and higher in saturated fats."*

Oh, no. Whenever you start bashing saturated fats, that's where you lose me. But the AHA tries to win back my confidence by saying:

> The benefits [of including fish in the diet twice a week] come from omega-3 fatty acids. While fish oil supplements are popular, the American Heart Association does not consider them a sufficient replacement for eating fish.

And they almost succeed. Supplements are not substitutes. The AHA and I are on the same page here (I can't believe I just wrote that...). Food is where most of us should get our nutrition. Expensive supplements can never bring balance to a cheap diet. Yet I'm not so sure I agree with the belief that omega-3s is why we all should be putting fish on our plates. After all, aren't omega-3s still a form of PUFAs?

Yes.

In fact, the ones found in fish are the longest chain versions of the PUFAs typically found in our diet. EPA is composed of twenty carbon atoms. DHA contains twenty-two. And with six double bonds, DHA earns the dubious distinction of most unsaturated of all the PUFAs. This means that any immunosuppressive, pro-inflammatory, anti-

---

*This idea is especially "true" if you either sell or manufacture the something in question.

thyroid effects attributable to the other polyunsaturated fatty acids are magnified when fish oil is used as a supplement.

See, all PUFAs are inherently fragile. As such, they are easily damaged, both in the manufacturing process as well as the digestive process. When exposed to light, heat, or oxygen—the very same things for which humans typically have an innate desire—PUFAs quickly become rancid, resulting in a large amount of free radical activity. Once set in motion, a chain reaction of destruction occurs until stopped by a sacrificial antioxidant. This is one reason why levels of vitamin E are so easily depleted when PUFAs are consumed—they are working to protect the body against lipid peroxidation (LPO). Left unchecked in the body, these free radicals act as carcinogens and readily damage arteries. Indeed, biopsies show that 74% of the fat found in clogged arteries is unsaturated, with 41% in the form of PUFAs. Additionally, advanced glycation end-products are toxic by-products formed when PUFAs react and bond to protein and sugar. Referred to, ironically, as AGEs, they are thought to be involved with accelerated aging and have been implicated in many chronic diseases.

I know this chapter is already getting way too long. Yet, I am nowhere near summarizing the many dangers of PUFAs, so I'll bullet point just a few more key points in case you still need convincing:

- PUFAs inhibit the action of proteolytic enzymes (involved in the digestion of food and the dissolving of blood clots).
- PUFAs damage the beta cells of the pancreas which produce and store insulin.
- PUFAs kill thymocytes (one of the numerous ways PUFAs compromise immunity).
- PUFAs lower mitochondrial activity and increases oxidative stress.
- PUFAs attenuate the production of testosterone.
- PUFAs keep sex steroid binding globulin (SSBG) from binding estrogen while also helping to activate the aromatase enzyme involved in the synthesis of estrogen. This contributes to estrogen dominance and its many manifestations.

The above list is by no means meant to be exhaustive. But I'm tired of writing about PUFAs, so I can imagine you're probably tired of reading about them. If that's the case, let me bring this subject to a close by emphasizing one final consideration. As the level of unsaturation increases, so does the propensity for the oil to have all the effects mentioned throughout this chapter.

And they don't get any more unsaturated than the ones sold as fish oil.

I know—I must be crazy! Speaking ill of fish oil is the equivalent of blasphemy in the field of nutrition.* But maybe it's time to listen to the heretics. You definitely can't rely on much of the research out there, especially if you don't know who funded it. But if you're looking for a truly unbiased view, I suggest using science as your source—true science has no agenda.

Lipid science shows that:

- *Marine oil's EPA/DHA spontaneously oxidizes at room temperature and more rapidly at normal body temperature—no level of antioxidants can stop this deleterious effect.*
- *Fish oil blunts the insulin response and raises resting blood glucose levels.*
- *Fish oil rapidly decreases arterial compliance—increasing "hardening of the arteries."*
- *Fish oil accelerates metastases in animals.*
- *Marine oil consumption impairs mitochondrial functionality, making it an anti-antiaging substance.*
- *Fish oil's EPA/DHA do nothing to increase cellular and tissue oxygenation; to the contrary, marine oils increase inflammation.*
- *The amount of EPA/DHA required by the brain is less than 7.2mg/day.*

In light of all the information presented in the previous pages, someone telling you to supplement with omega-3s from any source is a bit fishy, don't you think? And while I used to force cod liver oil down or swallow piles of omega fatty acid capsules, I just don't buy it anymore—literally or figuratively. Now, I believe the most prudent strategy when trying to counter the deleterious effects of an imbalanced Omega-3 to Omega-6 ratio or polyunsaturated fatty acids in general is to simply to minimize the amount of PUFAs in the diet in the first place.

---

http://www.ncbi.nlm.nih.gov/pubmed/16270286 is a link to some research my readers may find interesting. The authors of the study state: "Previously it was deduced that food rich in cholesterol and saturated fatty acids is atherogenic, while food rich in n-3 PUFAs was recognized to be protective against vascular diseases. These deductions are in contradiction to the fact that saturated fatty acids withstand oxidation while n-3 PUFAs are subjected to LPO like all other PUFAs.... Fish...contain besides n-3 PUFAs as minor constituents furan fatty acids (F-acids). These are radical scavengers and are incorporated after consumption of these nutrients into human phospholipids, leading to the assumption that not n-3 PUFAs, but F-acids are responsible for the beneficial efficiency of a fish diet."

I underlined part of the quote above for emphasis. LPO, if you'll note from the reference on the page before, is short for lipid peroxidation—a process best minimized if health is your goal.

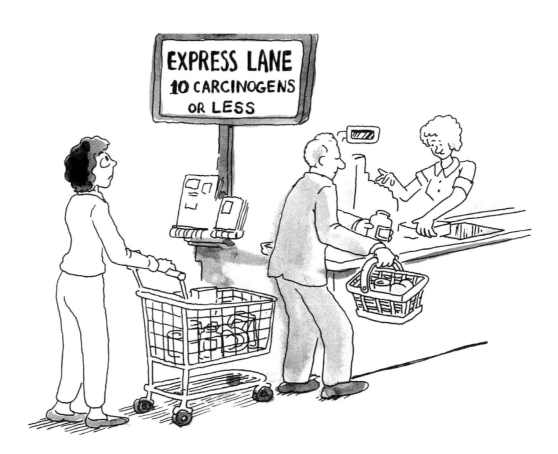

So what can I eat?

—Countless clients of mine

I cannot tell you the number of times my clients have pleaded with me to *"please, just tell me what the hell to eat!"* But I don't want to simply give them a fish. Having just finished the last chapter, you may think I'm not terribly inclined to teach them *how* to fish either. What I do want is for them (and you) to become self-sufficient. While keeping my clients dependent on me might be good for job security, it's really not the best business model. The problem here is twofold.

1) If I design a menu around food you don't like, you're either going to be hungry or completely unsatisfied—and likely both.
2) The more time I spend with you, the less time I'm able to spend with others who might benefit from working with me.

Besides, if you think the idea of someone telling you what to eat at *every* meal every day of your life sounds appealing, you're probably still living with your parents. In which case, I don't think you can afford to work with me.

But I am writing a book. Therefore, I appreciate the fact that many of my readers would benefit from a summary (and more elaboration, perhaps) of the nutritional recommendations thus far. So if your tastes require a bit more detail than the basic guidelines from Chapter One, below you will find an extensive list of foods divided into three different categories:

Optimal, Caution, and **Avoid**

I list them twice. The first time is for those who might simply want the information—an easy list to access when trying to tweak the diet in pursuit of health and performance. The second time I list the foods and include some information as to why these foods fall into their respective category. My experience has shown me that a person who understands the reasoning behind why certain actions are preferable over others is more likely to adhere to specific recommendations which may run contrary to their programming (not to mention contrary to conventional thinking).

OPTIMAL FOOD CHOICES

CARBOHYDRATES

FRUIT
- Apples
- Apricots
- Cherries
- Fresh Fruit Juices
- Grapefruit
- Nectarines
- Oranges
- Papaya
- Peaches
- Pears
- Pineapple
- Plums
- Tropical Fruit
- Watermelon

ABOVE GROUND VEGETABLES
- Cucumbers
- Peppers
- Squash
- Tomatoes
- Zucchini

BELOW GROUND VEGETABLES
- Beets
- Carrots
- Onions
- Potatoes
- Pumpkin
- Sweet potatoes
- Tubers

FATS
- Butter, from grass-fed sources
- Chocolate, dark with at least 70% cocoa content (and with no soy lecithin)
- Coconut Oil
- Cream, from grass-fed sources (and with no carrageenan)
- Olive Oil

PROTEINS
- Beef, grass-fed
- Bison, grass-fed
- Broth
- Cheese, no additives and from grass-fed sources
- Chicken, insect-fed/free-range
- Eggs, free-range
- Gelatin
- Goat
- Low-fat fish (e.g., cod, halibut, etc)
- Milk, from grass-fed sources
- Organ meat, grass-fed/free-range
- Pork, pastured
- Shellfish, wild
- Venison
- Yogurt, from grass-fed sources

CONSUME WITH CAUTION

CARBOHYDRATES

FRUIT
- Bananas, ripe with brown speckling and no green
- Berries
- Dried fruit
- Mango

BEANS AND LEGUMES
- Beans, soaked
- Legumes, soaked

GRAINS
- Buckwheat
- Cornmeal
- Ezekiel bread
- Millet
- Oats
- Quinoa
- Rice
- Sourdough
- Spelt

VEGETABLES
- Artichokes
- Asparagus
- Broccoli, well-cooked with saturated fat
- Brussel sprouts, well-cooked with saturated fat
- Cabbage, well-cooked with saturated fat
- Cauliflower, well-cooked with saturated fat
- Celery
- Eggplant
- Greens, well-cooked with saturated fat
- Mushrooms
- Peas

FATS
- Avocado
- Nuts, raw and soaked
- Nut butters
- Seeds, raw and soaked
- Seed butters

PROTEINS
- Eggs, conventional
- Grain-fed beef
- Grain-fed bison
- Grain-fed lamb
- Grain-fed pork
- Grain-fed poultry
- High-fat fish (e.g., salmon, tuna, etc)

AVOID AS POSSIBLE

ARTIFICIAL INGREDIENTS
- Basically anything you cannot pronounce or won't rhyme with something you'd read in a children's book

FOOD ADDITIVES
- Aspartame (now called AminoSweet)
- BHA and BHT
- Carrageenan
- Food color (e.g., red #40)
- Gums (e.g., guar, locust bean, xanthan, etc)
- Monosodium Glutamate (MSG)
- Nitrates
- rGBH (recombinant bovine growth hormone often used in dairy)
- Sodium benzoate
- Sucrolose
- Sulfur dioxide
- Synthetic vitamins (added to anything which is fortified)

FRIED FOODS
- Anything fried in an unsaturated fat

SOY PRODUCTS
- Soy lecithin
- Soy milk
- Soy protein
- Soy sauce

TRANSFATS
- Crisco
- Hydrogenated or partially hydrogenated oil
- Margarine and commercial butter substitutes

VEGETABLE OILS
- Canola
- Corn
- Cottonseed
- Grape seed
- Nut oils
- Peanut
- Sesame
- Safflower
- Soy
- Sunflower

OPTIMAL FOOD CHOICES

CARBOHYDRATES
FRUIT
- Apples (*Cooking will help break down the pectin, making them easier to digest. See the Resources section at the end of this book for my cooked apple recipe.*)
- Apricots
- Cherries
- Fresh Fruit Juices (*Pasteurized juices are devoid of enzymes, essentially making them less nutritious than non-pasteurized choices.*)
- Grapefruit (*Can impact the half-life of many pharmaceuticals, so use caution if currently taking certain medications.*)
- Nectarines
- Oranges
- Papaya
- Peaches
- Pears (*Cooking will help break down the pectin, making them easier to digest.*)
- Pineapple
- Plums
- Tropical Fruit
- Watermelon

ABOVE GROUND VEGETABLES—*These foods could easily be called "fruit-vegetables" as they tend to contain minimal amounts of PUFAs and are relatively low in the anti-nutrients common to most above ground vegetables.*
- Cucumbers
- Peppers
- Squash
- Tomatoes
- Zucchini

BELOW GROUND VEGETABLES—*The various threats these foods must protect themselves from are the same organisms that prey on humans, too. Bacteria, fungi, and parasites are the enemies these plants have learned to defend against. Thus, they are excellent sources of nutrition for humans and help protect our health when we consume them.*
- Beets (*Well-cooked and consumed with saturated fat.*)
- Carrots (*One medium sized raw carrot/day is an excellent defense against the buildup of endotoxins as well as preventing the absorption of excess estrogen—see the Resources section at the end of this book for an easy recipe for grated carrot salad.*)
- Onions
- Potatoes (*Well-cooked and consumed with saturated fat.*)
- Pumpkin
- Sweet potatoes (*Well-cooked and consumed with saturated fat.*)
- Tubers (*Well-cooked and consumed with saturated fat.*)

FATS

- Butter, from grass-fed sources
- Chocolate, dark with at least 70% cocoa content (and with no soy lecithin)
- Coconut Oil (*Refined will smell and taste less like coconut while also being more hypoallergenic than the unrefined versions. For more insights into the benefits of coconut oil, please refer to Chapter Nine.*)
- Cream from grass fed sources (and with no carrageenan)
- Olive Oil (*which passes the **PUFA test**—place the olive oil in the fridge & see if it starts to get cloudy. If it doesn't, PUFAs have been added.*)
- Palm Oil

PROTEINS

- Beef, grass-fed
- Bison, grass-fed (*U.S. bison, by definition, must be grass-fed.*)
- Broth (*See my simple recipe in the Resources section at the end of the book.*)
- Cheese, no additives and from grass-fed sources, preferably raw (*High levels of calcium in the diet help mitigate the mineral depleting effects of phytic acid. Raw dairy is preferable as pasteurization destroys essential enzymes in cheese like lactase which helps digest lactose. Additionally, many of the heat-sensitive nutrients are either damaged or destroyed. Raw cheeses are readily available in most grocery stores. Additionally, American consumers can find sources for raw dairy here at www.realmilk.com.*)
- Chicken, insect-fed/free-range
- Eggs, free-range (***NOTE*** *that eggs/chicken labeled as "free-range" in most if not all grocery stores really are not deserving of any health claims. Most are fed grains or soy. Unfortunately, chickens are not vegetarians; they are omnivores. As such, they cannot convert the PUFAs in their feed to saturated fat like ruminant herbivores can. This makes for sick chickens, poor quality eggs, and potential health issues for humans consuming them. Your best source will likely be a local farm or CSA which understands that chickens are more closely related to carnivorous dinosaurs than cows.*)
- Gelatin (*Make your own by using the bone broth recipe found in the Resources section at the end of this book or visit www.greatlakesgelatin.com.*)
- Goat
- Low-fat fish, wild not farmed (*Low-fat fish like cod, halibut, etc will be naturally lower in PUFAs compared to fattier fish.*)
- Milk, from grass-fed sources (*Pasteurization destroys essential enzymes in the milk like lactase which helps digest lactose. Enzymes are left intact in non-pasteurized products, which is why many people who are sensitive to dairy are able to tolerate raw milk or cheese. Additionally, many of the heat-sensitive nutrients are either damaged or destroyed. If you live in the United States, you can find sources for raw dairy here: www.realmilk.com.*)
- Organ meat, grass-fed/free-range
- Pork, pastured

- Shellfish, wild not farmed (*As with low-fat fish above, wild caught ensures the fish have not been exposed to antibiotics and pesticides common in the fish farming industry. Omega-6 content is higher in farmed fish as are levels of polychlorinated biphenyls or PCBs along with other toxins and chemical carcinogens.*)
- Venison
- Yogurt, from grass-fed sources

CONSUME WITH CAUTION

CARBOHYDRATES

FRUIT
- Bananas, ripe with brown speckling and no green (*Unripe bananas are high in starch, but you can allow time to make the sugars in the fruit more suitable for human digestion. And if they get overripe, freezing them for later use in a smoothie is always a possibility. See the Resources section at the end of this book for my typical smoothie recipe.*)
- Berries (*Seeds in the fruit can cause digestive issues and berries are also prone to mold.*)
- Dried fruit (*Can be high in mold and sulfites.*)
- Mango (*From the poison oak family and may cause reactions in sensitive people.*)

BEANS AND LEGUMES—*Beans contain PUFAs, mineral-binding phytates, and lectins. Some even contain phytohaemagglutinin (kidney beans are the worst offenders) which has known toxic effects resulting in severe gastrointestinal issues when consumed. Cooking reduces but does not eliminate these compounds and some studies have shown that heating at higher temperatures may actually potentiate these effects five-fold.*
- Beans, soaked
- Legumes, soaked (*Soaking is the traditional way of preparing these foods. Doing so will help eliminate phytic acid—an anti-nutrient found in these foods that inhibits the absorption of calcium, copper, iron, magnesium, and zinc. For more information, my readers may find the following article informative: http://nourishedkitchen.com/soaking-grains-nuts-legumes/*)

GRAINS—*All grains contain lectins and phytic acid as well as some level of PUFA (contributing approximately 33% of the linoleic acid and 25% of the alpha-linolenic acid intake in America). In addition, they are polysaccharides and can adversely impact blood sugar if not balanced effectively with the other macro nutrients. While the phytic acid content of most grains can be reduced by soaking them, the traditional method of preparation has little impact on the levels of this anti-nutrient in corn, millet, oats, or brown rice.*
- Buckwheat (*High in phytic acid and high on the glycemic index as well.*)
- Cornmeal (*Corn and its derivatives are naturally gluten free but also high in starch and likely genetically modified, so make sure to buy organic, cook well, and consume with a saturated fat.*)
- Ezekiel bread (*Sprouted grain, so the effects of phytic acid are mitigated. However, note that the bread still contains gluten.*)
- Millet (*While a non-gluten containing grain, millet is a goitrogen and will encourage thyroid inhibition. Indeed, while cooking often reduces the goitrogens found in foods, the reverse is true for this grain—it actually enhances the goitrogenic effect of millet.*)

- Oats (*Approximately half of people with gluten sensitivity will react to oats.*)
- Quinoa (*Closer to a seed than a grain, the outer coating of quinoa contains anti-nutrients called saponins. These substances readily increase the permeability of the small intestines, inhibiting nutrient delivery and increasing the uptake of foreign materials from which the gut would normally be protected.*)
- Rice (*White is best as many of the anti-nutrients are found predominately in the bran and germ portion of the grain.*)
- Sourdough (*The effects of phytic acid are mitigated, and even those who are gluten-sensitive will find they experience fewer digestive issues when consuming this type of bread.*)
- Spelt (*Often tolerated better than wheat, this ancient grain still contains gluten and is not suitable for people with celiac disease.*)

VEGETABLES
- Artichokes (*Cooking will help break down/soften the cellulose—refer to Chapter Nine.*)
- Asparagus (*Cooking will help break down/soften the cellulose—refer to Chapter Nine.*)
- Broccoli, well-cooked with saturated fat (*Eaten raw, this vegetable acts as a goitrogen and inhibits thyroid activity; also high in cellulose and PUFAs.*)
- Brussel sprouts, well-cooked with saturated fat (*Eaten raw, this vegetable acts as a goitrogen and inhibits thyroid activity; also high in cellulose and PUFAs.*)
- Cabbage, well-cooked with saturated fat (*Eaten raw, this vegetable acts as a goitrogen and inhibits thyroid activity; also high in cellulose and PUFAs.*)
- Cauliflower, well-cooked with saturated fat (*Eaten raw, this vegetable acts as a goitrogen and inhibits thyroid activity; also high in cellulose and PUFAs.*)
- Celery (*Cooking will help break down/soften the cellulose—refer to Chapter Nine.*)
- Eggplant (*Cooking will help break down/soften the cellulose—refer to Chapter Nine.*)
- Greens, well-cooked with saturated fat (*Eaten raw, these vegetables act as goitrogens and inhibit thyroid activity; they are also high in cellulose and PUFAs.*)
- Mushrooms (*Those with fungal issues may need to avoid mushrooms while healing.*)
- Peas (*More a fruit than a vegetable, peas are high in starch until cooked and/or allowed to mature.*)

FATS
- Avocado (*Higher in PUFAs than is optimal, avocado is best enjoyed as a garnish rather than a staple in the diet.*)
- Nuts, raw and soaked (*Nuts and seeds contain a smaller amount of phytic acid than grains. However, soaking them is still advised to help remove the high level of enzyme inhibitors. These substances work to keep the nut/see from sprouting prematurely but interfere with nutrient uptake and can*

cause digestive disorders. Raw is preferred as cooking, especially at higher temperatures, denatures the proteins and causes the unsaturated oils to become rancid. Also note that all nuts and seeds will have significant levels of PUFAs. Choosing types grown in tropical regions [e.g., macadamia] or minimizing the consumption of nuts and seeds altogether is recommended.)

- Nut butters
- Seeds, raw and soaked
- Seed butters

PROTEINS
- Eggs, conventional (*The food you are eating is condensing the nutrition or the toxins to which it was exposed. Thus, the grains or any other unsuitable substance fed to conventionally raised animals are in your diet "secondhand" when you choose to consume these foods.*)
- Grain-fed beef
- Grain-fed bison
- Grain-fed lamb
- Grain-fed pork
- Grain-fed poultry
- High-fat fish (*Salmon, tuna, etc are all high in PUFAs. And while much less of a health risk compared to fish/flax seed oil or any of the vegetable oils which are concentrated sources of PUFAs, these fish are best consumed in moderation to limit your intake of these unhealthy oils. Additionally, since fat attracts toxins, these fish typically have higher levels of chemicals and other carcinogens in their tissues than low-fat varieties. Minimizing high-fat fish in your diet will help minimize your exposure of these substances and the negative impact they can have on your health.*)

NOTE: Excess dietary phosphorus has been shown to adversely impact bone health secondary to high levels of parathyroid hormone (PTH). High PTH concentrations increase bone resorption. Some studies note that though "*increased Ca intake was beneficial for bone, as indicated by decreased S-PTH concentration and bone resorption....not even a high Ca intake could affect bone formation when P intake was excessive.*" (http://www.ncbi.nlm.nih.gov/pubmed/17903344/) Other studies indicated that "*higher Ca:P ratios contributed to a lower prevalence of central obesity.*" (http://www.ncbi.nlm.nih.gov/pmc/articles/PMC3702524/) Therefore, the consumption of large amounts of cereals, legumes, and flesh foods which are all high in phosphorus relative to calcium needs to be considered in the maintenance of a healthy diet.

AVOID AS POSSIBLE

ARTIFICIAL INGREDIENTS
- Basically anything you cannot pronounce or won't rhyme with something you'd read in a children's book

FOOD ADDITIVES—*Do I really need to elaborate on any of the items listed below?*
- Aspartame (*Now marketed under the brand AminoSweet, aspartame has resulted in more complaints to the FDA due to side affects than any other additive in FDA history.*)
- BHA and BHT (*Works to preserve your food. Sadly, it has the opposite effect on you. The National Toxicology Program concluded that BHA is "reasonably anticipated to be a human carcinogen" while the Center for Science in the Public Interest puts BHT on its "Caution" list.*)
- Carrageenan (*An indigestible polysaccharide derived from seaweed, carrageenan is consistently added to various foods as an emulsifier and thickening agent. Unfortunately, it has also been consistently used in experiments studying inflammation as it reliably produces an inflammatory response in test subjects. As research from an article in the 2001 edition of Environmental Health Perspective concluded "Because of the acknowledged carcinogenic properties of degraded carrageenan in animal models and the cancer-promoting effects of undegraded carrageenan in experimental models, the widespread use of carrageenan in the Western diet should be reconsidered."*)
- Food color (*Originally derived from coal tar but now from petroleum, these dyes are used by the food manufacturers primarily to keep costs down. Their safety, at best, is debatable. Many of these dyes have been proven to be carcinogenic in animals. DNA damage has also occurred. Additionally, consumption is highly correlated with ADHD as well as allergic reactions. And these conclusions are based off findings which studied only one dye at a time—strong consideration should also be given to when these dyes are consumed in combination. Natural dyes such as paprika or beet juice are healthier alternatives.*)
- Gums (*In short, guar gum, locust bean gum, xanthan gum, or any gum will gum up your intestines.*)
- Monosodium Glutamate (*MSG is a flavor enhancer. And if your food needs its flavor enhanced, perhaps you shouldn't eat it. Either way, the FDA granted it GRAS status. But with enough conflicting evidence about its safety—reactions ranging from "simple" headaches to possible damage of the hypothalamus—the FDA also requires it be listed on the ingredient list when it is added to a food.*)
- Nitrates (*This common preservative has been linked to many diseases from cancer to diabetes—all in the name of extending shelf life.*)
- rGBH (*Unless your cow is in a body building contest, I don't think it needs to be using recombinant bovine growth hormone.*)

- Sodium benzoate (*This or any other preservative is never good—the longer the shelf life of a food the shorter your life if you eat it.*)
- Sucrolose (*Sucrolose, sold under the trade-name of Splenda, is a man-made combination of chlorine and sugar or Chlorocarbon [though the manufacturers claim issue with this designation]. Chlorocarbons have long been known for causing organ, genetic, and reproductive damage and up to 40% shrinkage of the thymus, a gland that is the very foundation of our immune system. Sucralose also causes swelling of the liver and kidneys and calcification of the kidneys.*)
- Sulfur dioxide (*Another preservative given GRAS status, it can cause health problems in certain populations such as asthmatics or those sensitive to sulfites.*)
- Synthetic vitamins (*Anytime man tries to improve upon Mother Nature, we typically screw it up.*)

FRIED FOODS
- Anything fried in an unsaturated fat (*Hanging out with unstable people is potentially dangerous. Consuming foods fried in unstable fats is even worse.*)

SOY PRODUCTS (*Please see Chapter Eight [part II].*)
- Soy lecithin (*Besides being GMO, there's a high likelihood that any soy lecithin in your food will contain levels of pesticides and solvents as well as having some estrogenic activity.*)
- Soy milk (*If it doesn't have nipples, you shouldn't get milk from it. This rule applies to almond milk, rice milk, or any other dairy substitute.*)
- Soy protein (*An oxymoron as trypsin inhibitors in soy interfere with protein digestion.*)
- Soy sauce (*Most commercial soy versions are not fermented and should be avoided. Also, if not listed as organic, the soybeans used are likely GMO. Tamari is the only type of soy sauce made without wheat and is a better choice for those who are sensitive to gluten.*)

TRANS FATS
- Crisco (*Better known as trans fat in a can and quite possibly one of the largest contributors responsible for the rise of heart disease in America.*)
- Hydrogenated or partially hydrogenated oil (*Even though the FDA has made a preliminary determination that these oils are no longer "generally recognized as safe" and should eventually be phased out of the food supply, the USDA allows products with less than .5 grams of trans fat per serving to list the amount of trans fat on the label as 0 grams.*)
- Margarine and commercial butter substitutes (*There is no conspiracy theory among cows to give us all heart disease. Butter is better.*)

VEGETABLE OILS
- Canola (*29.6% PUFA*)
- Corn (*66% PUFA*)
- Cottonseed (*51.8% PUFA*)
- Grape seed (*70% PUFA*)
- Nut oils (*% of PUFA varies*)
- Peanut (*32% PUFA*)
- Safflower (*74.6% PUFA*)
- Sesame (*41.6% PUFA*)
- Soy (*57.8% PUFA*)
- Sunflower (*65.7% PUFA*)

My Typical Grocery List

Asparagus	Apples	Bacon	Butter
Beets	Bananas	Beef	Cheddar Cheese
Bell peppers	Blackberries	Bones	Cream
Carrots	Blueberries	Chicken	Half and Half
Celery	Cantaloupe	Duck	Parmigiano Reggiano
Cucumbers	Frozen Fruit	Fish	Sour Cream
Garlic	Kiwi	Hotdogs	Yogurt
Mushrooms	Lemon	Lamb	
Onions	Lime	Pork	Cocoa
Potatoes	Oranges	Sausage	Coconut Oil
Squash	Papaya	Shellfish	Ketchup
Sweet potatoes	Pears	1/4lb Bresaola	Olive Oil
Tomatoes	Pineapple	1/4lb Ham	Potato Flakes
Zucchini	Plums	1/3lb Salami	Sugar
	Prunes	1/2lb Turkey	Vinegar
	Raisins		
	Raspberries		
	Strawberries		
	Watermelon		

Enchilada Sauce	Beef Jerky	LOVE
Olives (with Anchovies)	Chocolate Chips	
Pickles	Dark Chocolate	
Rice Pasta	Fruit Roll Ups	
Rice	Honey	
Risotto	Ice Cream	
Sauerkraut	Jelly	
Soup	Juice Box	
Stewed Tomatoes	Orange Juice	
Taco Seasoning	Marshmallows	
Tomato Sauce	Tortillas	

In addition to the above items, we buy pastured eggs from a local farmer as well as raw milk (the latter is strictly for pet consumption should anyone with government ties happen to be reading this). So, yeah—we spend a *lot* of money on food, I guess. What can I say? I love to eat. I also love to be healthy. And I'd much rather spend money on my grocery bill than on my doctor's car payment.

You may notice that some of what we buy is on the *Consume with Caution* list. I'm just trying to be honest. I've never claimed to be infallible. I also believe that, given the right information, my family can make their own decisions as to what's right for them. By living 80% of the time with health in mind, their bodies are able to handle the 20% of the time they either can't make the best choice or maybe choose not to.

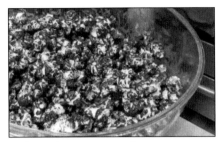

Now, personally, I may sometimes be a little closer to 90/10 or even 95/5, I'll admit. But outside of the **Avoid** list there's only one thing I know which is *never* included in my diet—deprivation.

(Chocolate covered popcorn is one of my favorite desserts.)

Here's an example of my weekly meals (often complimented with additional fruit based on my appetite). I did not include any of my sports nutrition for when I'm training or racing. Those specifics will be revealed in the Movement section of *Spot On.*

MONDAY:
—raspberry smoothie
—dark chocolate with blueberries
—corn tortilla with cheese and salsa (I often add leftover meat) and roasted veggies
—dried pineapple and raw cheddar cheese
—sword fish, rice, sautéed zucchini

TUESDAY:
—omelet with cheese, tomatoes, and onions and syrup or honey drizzled over it
—yogurt and chopped apples with gelatin and chocolate chips
—salad with beets, peppers, squash, turkey, cheese, and olives
—fresh squeezed orange juice with gelatin
—chicken and asparagus stir fry

WEDNESDAY:
—banana smoothie
—fried plantains and dark chocolate
—salad with cucumbers, carrots, tomatoes, feta, ham, balsamic vinegar
—parmigiano reggiano and raisins
—lamb chops and mashed sweet potatoes

THURSDAY:
—hash brown casserole with bacon, eggs, onions, and green peppers
—baked apple recipe
—butternut squash soup with feta
—spaghetti sauce with ground lamb over spaghetti squash
—honeydew melon and prosciutto

FRIDAY:
—left over spaghetti/spaghetti squash
—carrot salad recipe
—gluten free pizza with veggies
—bresaola with red peppers
—shrimp and cheese grits with sliced tomatoes

SATURDAY:
—strawberry smoothie
—dark chocolate with raspberries
—chicken wings/legs with mashed sweet potatoes and cranberries
—boiled eggs and carrots
—duck and fried potatoes

SUNDAY:
—pork sausage, gluten free pancakes, blueberries
—dates and parmigiano reggiano
—salad with cucumbers, carrots, tomatoes, feta, ham, balsamic vinegar
—plain yogurt with gelatin and raw cocoa powder
—pork ribs with roasted carrots and shallots

What about calories?

Yeah? What about them? I have no idea how many calories I eat, because I don't eat calories—I eat food. And now that you know which foods are optimal for human consumption, you probably won't need to be overly concerned with calories either. Simply put: health takes care of itself.

I tell my clients unless you're trying to win the Tour de France, counting calories is a colossal waste of time. Most foods worth eating don't come with a nutrition label anyway. Besides, did you know the United States Food and Drug Administration allows a 20% margin of error on the nutrition labels of foods? This means that 300 calorie *"meal replacement"* bar a person eats for lunch could pack an extra 60 calories which never get counted. And it doesn't take much for these little miscalculations to add up. Even if you're off by just an extra 100 calories a day—a mere 5% of what the Institute of Medicine holds is the average caloric need for a *sedentary* female adult—even then the impact could be huge. Over ten pounds in one year!

In my experience, however, many of the people having trouble with weight gain are actually not eating *enough*. The World Health Organization (WHO) defines hunger on their website, stating:

> *The energy and protein that people need varies according to age, sex, body size, physical activity and, to some extent, climate. On average, the body needs more than 2,100 kilocalories per day per person to allow a normal, healthy life. Extra energy is needed during pregnancy and while breast-feeding.*

In my practice, I consistently see new clientele trying to function on fewer than 1000 calories a day—technically a state of starvation. The record is a woman prescribed a 600 calorie diet by her General Practitioner in order to *"reset"* her metabolism. Oh, it reset her metabolism alright: back to the days of famines and plagues. She came in to my studio literally on fumes, dizzy from the Seesaw of Sickness. Her doctor didn't know shit about nutrition.

He didn't know anything about exercise either, but that didn't stop him from telling her she should "*do some cardio to accelerate her weight loss efforts.*" Yeah—go get your car. Fill up the tank only about one-third of the way. Then take off and drive it really fast. While you're at it, drive it really far, too. I don't care whose directions you follow or what your "mechanic" says. Sooner or later your trip's gonna end. And when it does, you'll need a hell of a lot more than a map to find the way back to health again.

Lack of fuel throws your biological machinery into the red. Challenge a system which is already under heavy load, and you risk breaking that system. Stress summates in the body. So, the greater your level of stress, the less your tolerance for exercise. These concepts are explained in more detail in the Movement section of *Spot On*. For now, just understand that, while it's not truly possible to be fat and healthy, it's all too easy to be skinny and sick. These days it's sadly all too simple. Follow a fad diet. Emulate reality weight-loss shows. Some of you may need go no farther than your doctor's office and ask for a prescription. Drastic diets or intense exercise or even fancy injections and supplements can all make you thin. Yet they can never make you healthy. True health is never extreme.

One of my nutrition mentors is a sweet, little woman in her seventies. She's about my height, weighs a bit less than me, and she does no formal exercise whatsoever. Any guesses as to how many calories she consumes a day? Come on—take a shot.

It's somewhere between 3000-3500 on average.

How is that even possible? No, she wasn't born with a fast metabolism. She just hasn't killed her metabolism like most of us do by dieting or over-exercising or eating foods not designed for human digestion—in essence, she hasn't starved herself. She hasn't lived her whole life in an energy crisis. She has a metabolism which works. It works because she's healthy. And she's healthy because it works.

The impact a given amount of food has on a person's physiology is predicated less on the total calories in that food and more on the total of what that person has done to themselves via nutrition and lifestyle choices. Your body is an incredibly accurate tool you can use to figure how best to fuel yourself... if you pay attention to it. And here's the best part—you get a new, updated version of that technology every morning you wake up.

There are some useful websites out there which can help you track your food. And I don't think it's a bad idea in the short term as it can prove very insightful when a person writes down what goes into his/her body. https://cronometer.com/ is one of the better ones. But the reason I like it has nothing to do with calories. If humans were nothing more than biological forms of the combustion engine—a view too often abused by the weight loss industry—calories in versus calories out might work. The focus on calories rather than nutrition is one of the reasons we're as sick as we are today.

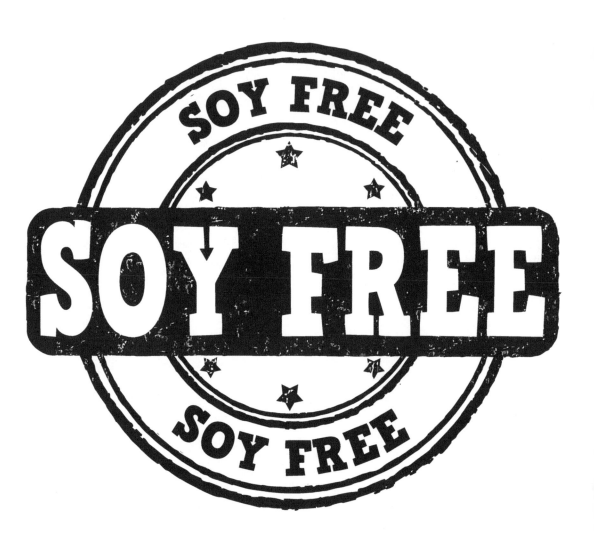

74

TOFU—soy bean curd, 1880, from Japanese tofu, from Chinese doufu, from dou "beans" + fu "rotten." Why does anybody eat this crap?

—Andrew Johnston's Twitter feed*

I got an e-mail from a friend of mine saying that, though she wasn't a vegetarian, her partner was. She said she wanted to include some sort of protein in the meals she cooked (it's good to have all the macronutrients represented on your plate) and was wondering what my thoughts on soy were.

Well, I used to think soy was the bomb! After all, the health claims surrounding soy were ubiquitous. You literally couldn't take a step without stepping in a claim—which, if you can pick up on my not-so-subtle analogy, you'll see what I now think of those advertisements. Because that's what they were: ads to convince people that soy is good for you. Now, have you ever seen a commercial for breathing? Breathing is good for you. So no one needs to do ads for it (though as our air gets worse, I'm sure those commercials are coming). Deprived of oxygen for three to four minutes, most people will die. Everyone knows this. What a lot of folks *don't* realize, however, is the more strongly something is marketed as being healthy for you, the worse it probably is for you.

Could it be possible a billion Chinese and Japanese folks actually have it wrong?

While it's true that the soybean first appeared during the Chou Dynasty (1134-246 BC), it did not become part of the Chinese menu for some time. Instead it was used in the process of crop rotation, fixing levels of nitrogen in the soil so that the Chinese could grow grains more suitable for human consumption like rice. Indeed, it wasn't until the Chinese discovered fermentation did soy, in the form of miso, tempeh, natto, and soy sauce, become widely consumed.

See, the Chinese knew that unfermented soybeans contain many different substances which make it unsuitable for human consumption. Foremost among these is phytic acid. Phytates block the absorption of calcium, copper, iron, magnesium, and zinc. So, even if your diet is rich in these nutrients, the consumption of soy can very easily lead to a deficiency in any one of them. All of these minerals are essential for health. Vegetarians who shun animal products like meat and diary and opt for soy to

---

*I love it when I can quote myself! And, no, I'm not narcissistic. It's just that at 5'4 my love of Self is highly concentrated.

"*replace*" this staple in the diet are, therefore, at a greater risk for a deficiency in any one of these nutrients.

Secondly, a large amount of trypsin and other enzyme inhibitors are present in soy blocking the absorption of these enzymes which are necessary for protein digestion. In tests, rats fed a diet of soy failed to grow normally. And everyone hates to see a malnourished rat...

Consuming soy that has been fermented lowers the levels of these anti-nutrients and makes items like miso, natto, and tempeh okay to eat. Tofu, on the other hand, has these anti-nutrients concentrated in the liquid and still present in the curd–thus its consumption is wrought with the same risks as soy in general. In truth, tofu isn't even fermented. It's actually precipitated, much like the process of making cottage cheese from milk. But if that makes tofu sound a bit more appealing, consider where the term tofu comes from: the Chinese word doufu–"dou" meaning beans and "fu" meaning rotten.

So how do the Chinese and Japanese stay so healthy on a diet so rich in soy? Well, maybe they don't eat as much as you thought. Eight grams/day in Japan and nine grams/day in China–that's less than two teaspoons. And while the Japanese do suffer less from some forms of cancer than here in America, cancer of the esophagus, liver, and stomach are much higher among the Japanese population than people in the U.S. Now that's a stat which should keep levels of patriotism healthy.

Healthy? That's what the United Soybean Program, which spends 80 million dollars a year to "*strengthen the position of soybeans in the marketplace and maintain and expand domestic and foreign markets for uses for soybeans and soybean products*" would like you to believe. 72 million acres of U.S. farmland is now devoted to soy, and it's one of the most highly pesticide-ridden crops grown today (and now genetically modified, too). Brazil, the second largest exporter of soy in the world next to the U.S., sacrifices millions of acres of rain forest to meet the demands of a growing number of people duped into eating isolated soy protein and textured vegetable protein for the reported health benefits.

Cholesterol lowering is one of these wonders. However, the "*benefits*" were only seen in individuals whose serum cholesterol levels were 250mg/dl or higher. And now that you know that cholesterol is actually protective, you might think differently about consuming anything which may cause those levels to drop.

In addition to being a major contributor of PUFAs in the Standard American Diet, soy is also high in isoflavones, a class of organic compounds and biomolecules related to flavonoids which act as phytoestrogens in mammals. These phytoestrogens, specifically genistein, are potent endocrine disruptors, causing infertility, reproductive problems, thyroid disease, and liver disease in test animals. But that's for animals in experiments which were fed an *extreme* amount of soy, right?? From an article by Sally Fallon:

Twenty-five grams of soy protein isolate, the minimum amount PTI claimed to have cholesterol-lowering effects, contains from 50 to 70 mg of isoflavones. It took only 45 mg of isoflavones in premenopausal women to exert significant biological effects, including a reduction in hormones needed for adequate thyroid function. These effects lingered for three months after soy consumption was discontinued.

One hundred grams of soy protein — the maximum suggested cholesterol-lowering dose, and the amount recommended by Protein Technologies International — can contain almost 600 mg of isoflavones, an amount that is undeniably toxic. In 1992, the Swiss health service estimated that 100 grams of soy protein provided the estrogenic equivalent of the Pill."

In fact, male children fed soy formula had reduced testicle size while female children experienced an earlier onset of puberty.* Alarming statistics like this prompted the New Zealand government in 1998 to issue a health warning about soy in infant formula. While animals on soy-based feed need supplementation with lysine for normal growth, the presence of soy in school lunch programs goes widely unnoticed (except by the wallets of the soy producers). A growing number of our children, therefore, may be at risk of the health consequences mentioned here and in countless other scientific publications and resources.

So what was my reply to my friend regarding preparing meals for her vegetarian partner? Get her to eat fish or meat. Tell her to consume dairy; or eat eggs or bone broth or anything.

Just say it isn't soy!

It might interest you to know that puberty is related to longevity, with later onset indicative of longer lifespan in animals.

SOY DANGERS SUMMARIZED:

- High levels of phytic acid in soy reduce assimilation of calcium, magnesium, copper, iron and zinc. Phytic acid in soy is not neutralized by ordinary preparation methods such as soaking, sprouting and long, slow cooking. High-phytate diets have caused growth problems in children.

- Trypsin inhibitors in soy interfere with protein digestion and may cause pancreatic disorders. In test animals, soy containing trypsin inhibitors caused stunted growth.

- Soy phytoestrogens disrupt endocrine function and have the potential to cause infertility and to promote breast cancer in adult women.

- Soy phytoestrogens are potent anti-thyroid agents that cause hypothyroidism and may cause thyroid cancer. In infants, consumption of soy formula has been linked to autoimmune thyroid disease.

- Vitamin B_{12} analogs in soy are not absorbed and actually increase the body's requirement for B_{12}.

- Soy foods increase the body's requirement for vitamin D.

- Fragile proteins are denatured during high temperature processing to make soy protein isolate and textured vegetable protein.

- Processing of soy protein results in the formation of toxic lysinoalanine and highly carcinogenic nitrosamines.

- Free glutamic acid or MSG, a potent neurotoxin, is formed during soy food processing and additional amounts are added to many soy foods.

- Soy foods contain high levels of aluminum which is toxic to the nervous system and the kidneys.

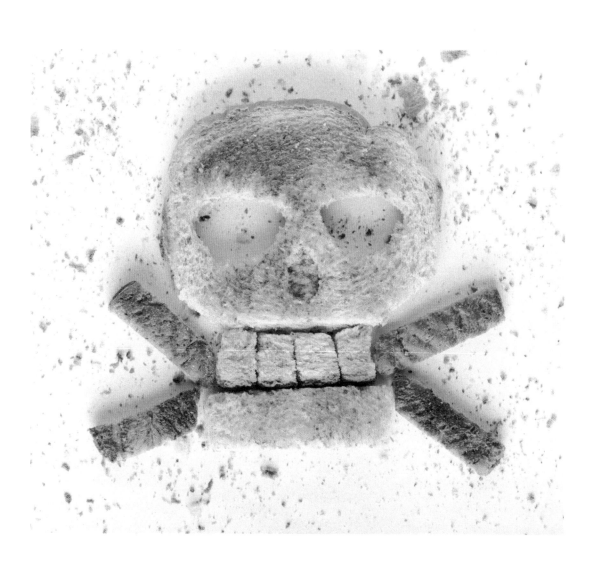

Andrew,

I just had to write to you and tell you how great I am feeling. I am trying to not be dramatic when I say that going gluten free is changing my life. I feel SO much clearer headed and have an outrageous amount of energy. I can't stop cleaning and organizing things. This has NEVER been my idea of fun. I feel almost as if I have had an awakening. So excited to see what happens next! Just thought you would like to know.

—another satisfied client of mine

Biohealth Diagnostics estimates that 60% of Caucasians have gluten sensitivity. Many experts out there will tell you that it's as high as 90% of white skinned people with other races close behind. Unfortunately, most gluten intolerance tests fail to screen for antibodies to beta-gliadin, gamma-gliadin, omega-gliadin, or transglutaminase 3 & 6. So even though the 2003 edition of the Archives of Internal Medicine report that only 1 in 133 has full blown Celiac Disease, countless others are needlessly suffering because their symptoms have been *"proven"* to be unrelated to diet.

I'm here to tell you that one of the most reliable signs that you may be gluten intolerant is if you have opposable thumbs and know what Facebook is.

When a person is sensitive to gluten, ingesting any grain other than rice, buckwheat, millet, or corn will inflame the gut wall. This microtrauma to the intestine causes tiny holes to form, allowing food particles to pass into the bloodstream undigested. The body then creates antibodies to that particular food, potentially causing you to have an immune response to whatever you're eating. This means that the bloating, the gas, the diarrhea, or any other digestive disorders you've experienced due to gluten consumption, you'll now have with almost any food in your diet.

As a case in point, a few years ago I began coaching a guy who presented with a host of symptoms I believed might be related to what he was eating. The ten day food log I require of all clients before I will work with them showed he had the same breakfast every morning—a bagel and eggs. Of course, there were a lot other areas in need of improvement, but I didn't want to overwhelm him. So I suggested he consider taking gluten out of his diet for a bit. I'm not sure if it was my style of coaching or if he thought farting every third step was normal, but he told me he didn't have any issue with gluten. Even though he probably wasn't truly clear on what gluten is, he told me he'd *"eaten gluten all his life with no problems."*

Now, when you have a diet of clean, life-giving foods, free of chemical additives and preservatives, eating anything different is going to be immediately noticeable. Of

81

course, the reverse is true, too. A diet of processed crap you can barely digest won't seem much different when you add some artificial, man-made junk to your plate. It was obvious this guy's personal experience with health kept him blind to many of his body's signals, so I asked him to do what's called a bloodspot test—a simple procedure which would give him quantifiable evidence of how his body was responding to certain foods. He agreed. Unfortunately, while we were waiting for results, he heard about the so-called *"Master Cleanse"* and decided to give that a shot, too.

If you've never head of this particular fast, the Master Cleanse involves consuming nothing but a homemade combination of water, maple syrup, cayenne pepper, and lemon juice. I have to applaud my client for his will power—he consumed nothing but this concoction for ten whole days before we got back together to discuss the findings of his bloodspot test which showed he was, indeed, gluten intolerant. The results also indicated he was becoming sensitive to a lot of other random foods which aren't typically a problem for most people: asparagus; lettuce; beef—in all, he was having issues with twelve usually benign foods. Yet, instead of being alarmed, my client started questioning the validity of the test, saying he felt no better despite being *"gluten free for over a week!"* I suppressed a strong urge to go off on one of my soapbox sermons and calmly suggested we repeat the test. He agreed, albeit reluctantly. When the results came back the second time, gluten was still on the list.

But now so were cayenne pepper, maple syrup, and lemon....

My client's gut was leaking worse than a rusty sieve. On the bright side, those openings in his intestines at least helped open his eyes. His objective mind finally had the proof it needed to realize his digestive system was a hot, smoldering mess. Now that he could sense the smoke, I knew I could convince him he had to put out the fire.

Chronic inflammation in the gut causes what's termed villous atrophy. Lining the wall of your intestines, you have little finger like projections called villi. These, in turn, have tiny little microvilli covering them—you have about 200 million per square millimeter. The job of the microvilli is to help you assimilate nutrition from your food by producing various enzymes. Unfortunately, with villous atrophy, the gut wall gets blasted and the intestine end up looking barer than Old Mother Hubbard's cupboard. Less surface area = less micro villi = less nutrient absorption. This leads people down the road of sickness and obesity as they're forced to eat more to maintain nutrient status.

Now, like my client in the scenario above, many of the people with whom I consult will swear they don't have a problem with gluten. *"How could I? We've been eating bread for eons,"* they'll say, *"so how can it be bad for us?"*

Well, for starters—the human genus, *Homo*, has been on this earth for some 2,000,000 years or more. Yet grains only entered our diet during the agricultural revolution which began approximately 10,000 years ago. Since research shows it takes the human genome 100,000 years to change 1/10th of one percent, our history of farming grains is a flash in the pan as far as human evolution is concerned. But even if some of us have somehow developed the digestive capacity early members of the grain lobby would have praised, the fact is that ain't your grandma's bread you're eatin' anymore! Fifty years ago, wheat contained only 5% gluten. Today it's as high as 50%.

Perhaps a more important point to consider is there probably wasn't a whole lot of glyphosate being sprayed on wheat back then either. *Roundup* is the world's most popular herbicide. During 2007 in the U.S. alone, 185 million pounds of it was applied to a variety of crops including wheat. Though considered "safe" by both Monsanto—the manufacturer—and the EPA, the use of Roundup is nothing if not controversial. It has been linked to variety of health disorders. Most notable in regards to our current discussion, it has been implicated in the increasing incidence of Celiac Disease. Below you can find an excerpt from a study entitled *Glyphosate, pathways to modern diseases II: Celiac Sprue and Gluten Intolerance* by Anthony Samsel and Stephanie Seneff:

> *Celiac disease, and, more generally, gluten intolerance, is a growing problem worldwide, but especially in North America and Europe, where an estimated 5% of the population now suffers from it. Symptoms include nausea, diarrhea, skin rashes, macrocytic anemia and depression. It is a multifactorial disease associated with numerous nutritional deficiencies as well as reproductive issues and increased risk to thyroid disease, kidney failure and cancer. Here, we propose that glyphosate, the active ingredient in the herbicide, Roundup® is the most important causal factor in this epidemic. Fish exposed to glyphosate develop digestive problems that are reminiscent of celiac disease. Celiac disease is associated with imbalances in gut bacteria that can be fully explained by the known effects of glyphosate on gut bacteria. Characteristics of celiac disease point to impairment in many cytochrome P450 enzymes, which are involved with detoxifying environmental toxins, activating vitamin D_3, catabolizing vitamin A, and maintaining bile acid production and sulfate supplies to the gut. Glyphosate is known to inhibit cytochrome P450 enzymes. Deficiencies in iron, cobalt, molybdenum, copper and other rare metals associated with celiac disease can be attributed to glyphosate's strong ability to chelate these elements. Deficiencies in tryptophan, tyrosine, methionine and selenomethionine associated with celiac disease match glyphosate's known depletion of these amino acids. Celiac disease patients have an increased risk to non-Hodgkin's lymphoma, which has also been implicated in glyphosate exposure. Reproductive issues associated with celiac disease, such as infertility, miscarriages, and birth defects, can also be explained by glyphosate. Glyphosate residues in wheat and other crops are likely increasing recently due to the growing practice of crop desiccation just prior to the harvest. We argue that the practice of "ripening" sugar cane with glyphosate may explain the recent surge in kidney failure among agricultural workers in Central America. We conclude with a plea to governments to reconsider policies regarding the safety of glyphosate residues in foods.*

While there may be numerous reasons to limit wheat in the diet, the above abstract from the November 2013 issue of *Interdisciplinary Toxicology* has to be one of the most damning. Or maybe it's just a mark against using any grains that aren't organic—which in the United States, at least, is the majority of what's consumed. If that's the case, then perhaps the problems associated with cereals, breads, and pastas are simply more an issue of accumulation. Could it be that when modern-day food manufacturing practices are coupled with the heavy use of chemical pesticides and fertilizers found in conventional farming it's enough to make grains an intolerable burden on human health? The dietary straw which breaks our digestive back?

I'll admit—whether it's gluten or left over chemical residue or something else entirely—uncovering the true etiology of the symptoms requires a bit of detective work. Average retention time in the healthy human body is 56-72 hours. This means you can consume something which you're sensitive to on Monday and not have a reaction until Thursday. Thus, it can be almost impossible for you to put two and two together, especially if your bowels are so destroyed you're constantly going number three.

So how do you correlate cause with effect? My suggestion as far as gluten is concerned is to remove all potential sources from your diet for at least two weeks and see how you feel. Thirty days would be better. Sixty days would be ideal as it takes, on average, about two months for the gut wall to *begin* to heal. Yet, a lot of people will have a very hard time with this approach as they are literally addicted to gluten. Or more specifically, they're addicted to the dopamine created to counter the pain of an inflamed intestinal wall. Fortunately, they'll often notice a marked increase in energy and vitality if they can at least last a good two weeks. And there might be some intended consequences, too.

I started working with a pretty good cyclist a few years back. He was as thin as he was tall—I had to get on a step stool to perform some of my tests during his physical assessment if that tells you anything—yet, he had a noticeable paunch you wouldn't have expected from someone so lean. I looked at him and immediately knew he was gluten intolerant. When you've been in the business as long as I have, you can look at some people and just tell. I asked if he'd be willing to try a gluten-free diet, telling him I thought it would improve his power-to-weight ratio. He did, and his body responded exactly like I had expected except for one surprise: all the cracks on his heels also disappeared. See, for as long as he could remember the skin there was dry and constantly irritated. He'd seen dermatologist after dermatologist; he'd tried every cream and ointment on the market, but his heels were always painful, even bleeding at times. Yet, in just two months of emancipation from gluten his feet looked normal again.

Estimates hold that more than half of patients diagnosed with what's called Non-Celiac Gluten Sensitivity have no symptoms of gastrointestinal dysfunction. I don't know how many of these folks suffer from ugly feet, but statistics show neurological disorders such as pain or numbness account for approximately 10% of complaints. Impaired cognitive function is so common among those sensitive to gluten it has become known as *"grain brain"* with a book of the same title becoming a *New York Times* bestseller. Less well known (and maybe because there's no accompanying cook book to sell) is a study from 1976 entitled *Wheat gluten as a pathogenic factor in schizophrenia*. The authors write:

> *Schizophrenics maintained on a cereal grain-free and milk-free diet and receiving optimal treatment with neuropleptics showed an interruption or reversal of their therapeutic progress during a period of "blind" wheat gluten challenge. The exacerbation of the disease process was not due to variations in neuroleptic doses. After termination of the gluten challenge, the course of improvement was reinstated. The observed effects seemed to be due to a primary schizophrenia-promoting effect of wheat gluten.*

Many other studies have reached similar conclusions:

> *A drastic reduction, if not full remission, of schizophrenic symptoms after initiation of gluten withdrawal has been noted in a variety of studies.* http://www.ncbi.nlm.nih.gov/pubmed/16423158

> *Clinical manifestations in patients with NCGS are characteristically triggered by gluten and are ameliorated or resolved within days to weeks of commencing a gluten-free diet. Emerging scientific literature contains several reports linking gluten sensitivity states with neuropsychiatric manifestations including autism, schizophrenia, and ataxia.* http://www.ncbi.nlm.nih.gov/pubmed/24693281

> *... gluten sensitivity remains undertreated and underrecognized as a contributing factor to psychiatric and neurologic manifestations.* http://www.ncbi.nlm.nih.gov/pubmed/21877216

I know—it all sounds implausible! But did you know that the gut has its own nervous system? It's called the Enteric Nervous System (ENS). Separate from the Central Nervous System (CNS), the ENS is formed early in embryonic development and later connects to the CNS via the vagus nerve. With some 100,000 neurons, at least as many as is contained in the entire length of the spinal cord, this branch of your nervous system is critical as it actually has the capacity to both learn and to remember. The *"gut feeling"* some people get is one example of this phenomenon. Research shows the ENS greatly influences your energy levels, tolerance for exercise, even your mood. Thus, diet literally impacts not only a person's physiology but his/her *psychology*, as well. In fact, a doctor named Byron Robinson thought the ENS was so important that he dedicated an entire book on the subject entitled *The Abdominal and Pelvic Brain*. First published over one hundred years ago, the book is a bit dated now. After all, since most people treat their gut like a garbage can, a more appropriate title these days would be *The Abdominal and Pelvic Landfill*. Still, some of his observations are especially pertinent to our current state of health:

"In mammals there exist two brains of almost equal importance to the individual and race. One is the cranial brain, the instrument of volitions, of mental progress and physical protection. The other is the abdominal brain, the instrument of vascular and visceral function. It is the automatic, vegetative, the subconscious brain of physical existence. In the cranial brain resides the consciousness of right and wrong. Here is the seat of all progress, mental and moral...However, in the abdomen there exists a brain of wonderful power maintaining eternal, restless vigilance over its viscera. It presides over organic life. It dominates the rhythmical function of viscer...The abdominal brain is a receiver, a reorganizer, an emitter of nerve forces. It has the power of a brain. It is a reflex center in health and disease...The abdominal brain is not a mere agent of the [cerebral] brain and cord; it receives and generates nerve forces itself; it presides over nutrition. It is the center of life itself. In it are repeated all the physiologic and pathologic manifestations of visceral function (rhythm, absorption, secretion, and nutrition). The abdominal brain can live without the cranial brain, which is demonstrated by living children being born without cerebrospinal axis. On the contrary the cranial brain can not live without the abdominal brain..." (Robinson, 1907, pp. 123 -126)*

Read Robinson's last comment again: *"the cranial brain can not live without the abdominal brain."* In light of that insight, how important do you think it is we take the time to become cognizant of what we put in our mouths? Think about what you eat, because what you eat can be quite literally what and how you think! If the diet of a person fails to support gut health, it can in no way hope to support mental and emotional health either.

Here, then, the studies of Weston A. Price in nutrition along with Paul Maclean and the Triune Brain come together to both complement and support Robinson's work with the enteric nervous system. Medical doctors have been slow to take notice. Or, perhaps, it would be more accurate to say they've often been too quick to dismiss what traditional cultures have known for generations. But as Confucius said, *"Three things cannot long be hidden: the sun, the moon, and the truth."* And as we become more adept at trusting our gut instincts instead of waiting for Western Medicine to finally see though their double blind studies, we can once again take charge of our own vitality.

A simple first step in achieving such a lofty goal may be as easy as giving up gluten. That small change, however, ultimately requires serious commitment. I usually tell people that the folks out there espousing an *"all or nothing"* approach don't know it all (which should give you an idea as to what they *really* know). In the case of gluten sensitivity, however, a strategy of strict avoidance is the only practical choice. As little as *one gram* of gluten can create an immune response in the body, so you literally have to cut it out completely to reap the benefits. I actually think it's a good idea to avoid all grains in the short-term. Most contains proteins which are similar enough to gluten to elicit an immune response. Nuts and seeds or any food high in phytates can also cause reactions in sensitive people, so I suggest eliminating these foods, too (besides, they're on the *Consume with Caution* list...).

Livingwithout.com is a great resource for you as you evolve into a gluten free diet. The site provides good tips and tasty recipes as you navigate a world without wheat. And you really have to be careful with ingredients as some potential sources of gluten which may surprise you include:

- Alcohol made from grains
- Artificial color
- Battered or fried anything
- Bouillon
- Emulsifiers
- Grain-fed meats, dairy, eggs, or even farm-raised fish
- Gravy
- Hydrolyzed or textured protein
- Mayonnaise
- Modified food starch
- MSG
- Natural flavors
- Non-dairy creamer
- Salad dressing
- Soy sauce
- Stabilizers
- Vinegar (unless it specifically states wine vinegar or balsamic vinegar, etc)

Most of that junk you are hopefully now avoiding anyway. The Food Allergen Labeling and Consumer Protection Act of 2004 currently requires foods or ingredients which contain or are derived from wheat clearly state so on the label. But I still think it's a good idea to become a gluten detective rather than relying on the food manufacturers or the USDA to have your back.

So in conclusion, if you want to be healthy, simply don't follow the herd. In fact, move 180 degrees opposite of everyone else. Swim against the stream and you'll probably be moving in the right direction. Indeed, I think the best advice I could give anyone is to go against the grain! Because the truth is—if you have a digestive or neurological disorder of unknown origin & you're still eating a bunch of bread, cereal, and pasta, you're really nothing but a gluten* for punishment.

*We can't just blame wheat—not if we're being honest. In addition to foods we may be intolerant of, the usual suspects responsible for a leaky gut include alcohol, medicinal drugs, and stress. It's our lifestyle. And you control that! So it's a good thing you're reading Spot On as its contents will help you take responsibility for yourself.

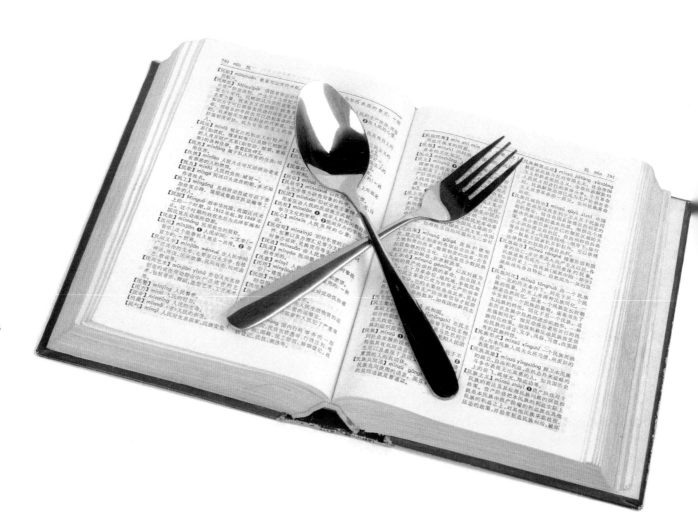

CHAPTER NINE

At the potluck, I brought two dishes: knowledge and mashed potatoes and gravy. Guess which one got cleaned out and which one hardly got touched.

—Jarod Kintz

Earlier in this section, in Chapter Three, I wrote that the terms in bold from the *Seesaw of Sickness* would be explained in more detail. Since my business model of under promising and over delivering has served me pretty well during my career, I'm now going to elaborate on those terms along with several select others. Everyone's appetite for knowledge is different, however. So take from the ones you want and skip the ones you don't care for; I won't be offended either way. I simply enjoy feeding your healthy curiosity—and your health.

When **Energy Production** *goes down,* **Adrenaline** *goes up.*
When **Adrenaline** *goes up,* **Intestinal Circulation** *(of glucose and O_2) goes down.*
When **Intestinal Circulation** *goes down,* **Endotoxin Production** *goes up.*
When **Endotoxin Production** *goes up,* **Liver Function** *goes down.*
When **Liver Function** *goes down,* **Toxic Load** *goes up.*
When **Toxic Load** *goes up,* **Energy Production** *goes down.*

Energy Production—basically, we're talking about metabolism here. Without a healthy metabolism, you cannot be healthy...as Ray Peat says *"oxidative metabolism is about 15 times more efficient than the non-oxidative 'glycolytic' or fermentive metabolism; higher organisms depend on this high efficiency oxidation for maintaining integration and normal functioning."* You are one of these *"higher organisms"*, so treat your body accordingly!

Adrenaline—made in the adrenals, this hormone often acts in concert with cortisol to increase blood sugar, by utilizing the body's own tissues. Indeed, any stress—from over exercise to under eating—is considered by the body as a need for blood sugar in order to run the various biological systems necessary for either fight or flight. Unfortunately, the mobilization of the body's adipose tissues increases the cells' exposure to PUFA as the oxidation of glucose is inhibited. This causes a slowdown of energy production which further stimulates the production of adrenaline and the other stress hormones in a positive feedback loop. Increased fat oxidation results in less CO_2 being produced which then impairs O_2 delivery in the body. Additionally, both intestinal health as well as intestinal functioning are compromised as blood is shunted to the working muscles and away from what—at the time—is considered non-essential bodily functions.

Intestinal Circulation—the intestines can only function optimally when blood flow allows critical nutrients to be delivered. If circulation is compromised for any reason, both digestion and elimination slow down or cease, creating an ideal environment for the proliferation of different pathogens that can cause various health issues. Poor circulation can also be the catalyst for *"leaky gut syndrome"* as the walls of the intestines lose their barrier function and become more permeable to undigested food particles, endotoxins, and other dangerous substances.

Endotoxin Production—also known as lipopolysaccharides or LPS, endotoxins are strong bacterial poisons that are always present within the intestines of otherwise healthy humans. A well-functioning liver prevents normal levels of LPS from becoming systemic. However, when bacterial concentrations increase secondary to compromised motility from food sensitivities or other lifestyle factors (e.g., exercise—see the Movement section in *Spot On*), endotoxin can overburden and even injure the liver. Hepatic damage creates a vicious cycle wherein LPS continue to accumulate causing further liver dysfunction. Another side effect of endotoxin is it inhibits glucoronidation—a step in Phase II detoxification occurring in the liver during which estrogen and other potential health threats are neutralized and cleared from the body.

Liver Function—the liver weighs in at approximately three pounds in the adult human. The largest gland in the body, it is involved in hundreds of essential biological functions, the most important of which is, arguably, detoxification. Toxins in the form of alcohol, drugs, and other harmful substances—including PUFA—are prepared for excretion via urine or feces as long as the liver remains healthy and well-nourished. It is also responsible for the clearance of various *"used"* hormones including estrogen. In addition, the liver produces bile to aid in the digestion of fats; it stores glycogen and converts it to glucose as the need arises; and it's a reservoir for several vitamins including A, D, B_{12}, and K as well as a storage site for iron.

Toxic Load—the onslaught of chemicals, pharmaceuticals, pollutants, and even the body's own metabolic byproducts continually challenge the liver and the other organs of detoxification. When the various systems of the body are all running efficiently, clearance rate of these various toxins is adequate to maintain homeostasis under normal conditions. A healthy metabolism is the one pre-requisite for this to occur.

Adrenocorticotropic Hormone (ACTH)—ACTH is a corticotropic hormone made in the pituitary gland under the direction of the hypothalamus. It stimulates the release of cortisol and (to a lesser degree) influences the production of aldosterone.

Aldosterone—a steroid hormone, aldosterone is part of the rennin-angiotensin-aldosterone system (RAAS). Stimulated by increased plasma concentrations of potassium, it raises blood pressure, retains both sodium and water, and influences the release of cortisol. Recently, aldosterone has also bee recognized as a common feature in depression (note the entry under *Serotonin* below).

Cellulose—the polysaccharide found in the cell walls of all types of plants, giving them structure, rigidity, and support, cellulose is considered the most abundant organic compound on earth. It is found in the human diet primarily in the form of vegetables and fruits. Since we do not produce cellulases—enzymes that break down the cellulose molecule into monosaccharides—cellulose is considered an insoluble fiber and passes through the human digestive system without being absorbed, providing no calories or vitamins and minerals. Its nutritional value, reportedly, comes from the fact that it provides bulk to our stools, providing a stimulus that triggers peristalsis in the intestines.

A tire tread from an eighteen-wheeler left on the side of the highway is also indigestible. Chop it up into bite-size pieces and have it for lunch, and I'm pretty sure it's gonna do more than bulk up your stool. Of course, if that analogy is bit too far-fetched for your imagination, then think about eating something more natural—like a bunch of cotton, say. At approximately 90% cellulose, that's not going to be digested all that well either. Wood is only 40-50% cellulose. But unless you're a termite, I think you'll still need a chaser to get it out the other end—something like Drano, perhaps.

The point I'm trying to make is that roughage can be rough on the system. Gas, bloating, diarrhea—all these are signs of poor digestion. Yet these complaints are also common side effects of a high-fiber diet. They'd probably be side effects of munching on Michelins, too. As the history of modern-day food processing shows, however, people will put up with just about any digestive complaint if they are convinced something is healthy. Ray Peat writes that "*almost anything becomes 'food' when people are under economic and social pressure.*" I don't know if white-walled radials would qualify, but cellulose has definitely received its share of praise in scholarly articles. Consider this statement from a 2010 paper, which appeared in the journal *Nutrients*:

> *The digestive and viscosity characteristics of dietary fiber are the likely modes of action which affect diabetes and obesity risk.*

Plenty of "*research*" supports the hypothesis that fiber facilitates weight loss and contributes to health. Unfortunately, I would say these same studies often perpetuate the idea that losing weight and being healthy are synonymous. And nothing could be further from the truth.

I remember a bike race I did in an absolute downpour somewhere in Spain. The spray coming off the tires in front of me got in my eyes, my nose, my mouth. By the time I reached the finish line, I literally had a taste of the Spanish countryside. And, as I was about to find out, one of the flavors I had been treated to was the chicken shit which covered most of the roads in that particular region.

The night after the race I was trapped inside the bathroom of our small, third floor apartment fighting desperately with my colon. My wife and I had been together for over seven years without me so much as farting in front of her (though she admits she

91

let one go on our first date and blamed it on my dog). So my bowels were as well-trained as my quads. But as I held onto the toilet like it was a bucking bronco, the sounds leaking past the door left nothing to the imagination. Random explosions of body fluids roared into the toilet. A continual barrage of alternating deep and high-pitched guttural spurts escaped through our paper thin walls, eventually waking my wife who came to see if I was okay. In between the sporadic gunshots flying out of my backside and ricocheting off the inside of the toilet bowl, I begged her desperately not to come in. It wasn't my pride so much as my worry the smell might overwhelm her if she opened the door. At the very least, I didn't want to risk the memory of my stench threatening our martial union.

When the attack ended, and my body had finally vanquished the last remnants of whatever had laid siege to my intestines, I climbed off the toilet like a weak old man. You could probably find a scale like the one I immediately stepped on in any professional cyclist's bathroom. 112lbs—eleven pounds lighter than my normal racing weight. I half smiled and thought about how fast I could probably go uphill now. My delirium kept me from recognizing the absolute insanity of that idea. And my wife, thankfully, kept me from riding by bike until I was strong enough to actually get out of bed.

Any fool can lose weight. Only the wise can be truly healthy.

Am I saying that my precipitous drop in weight mirrored my I.Q.? Well, that's (somewhat) debatable. What is beyond argument is that all systems of the body, including the one that runs elimination, require a healthy metabolism to work efficiently. Yet, consider an excerpt from the exact same paper quoted above:

The digestive and viscosity characteristics of dietary fiber....appear to decrease nutrient absorption, therefore, decreasing metabolizable energy.

It's right there in black and white—dietary fiber decreases nutrient absorption and energy! Well that'll get the Seesaw of Sickness cranked up! Since in many cases we're already so unhealthy in the first place, decreased energy production simply keeps that seesaw going. Indeed, while I think it's obvious that *excessive* consumption of high cellulose containing foods can inhibit health via a number of different ways (including irritating the gut and the subsequent release of serotonin as noted below), I want to emphasize a critical element which is too often ignored. If someone's metabolism is already compromised, for whatever reason, that person's capacity to consume high cellulose foods without ill effects is severely limited. When health is not sufficient to support the normal functioning of all the body's systems—especially digestion—then eating a bunch of salads or raw vegetables or any high-fiber food is the worst thing you can do. Again, as Ray Peat writes:

Polysaccharides and oligosaccharides include many kinds of molecules that no human enzyme can break down, so they necessarily aren't broken down for absorption until they encounter bacterial or fungal enzymes. In a well maintained digestive system, those organisms will live almost exclusively in the large intestine, leaving the length of the small intestine for the absorption of monosaccharides without fermentation. When digestive secretions are inadequate, and peristalsis is sluggish, bacteria and fungi can invade the small intestine, interfering with digestion and causing inflammation and toxic effects.

Or if I may put it in an Andrewism you can more easily remember: *cellulose=cell-u-lose.*

Essential Fatty Acids (EFA): Alpha-Linolenic Acid (ALA) and Linoleic Acid (LA)—fats which mainstream medicine (note, I didn't say *"nutrition"*) considers essential because the human body does not synthesize them. The human body also doesn't make arsenic or cyanide, either, but maybe that's beside the point. What our bodies *do* make is Mead Acid—an unsaturated n-9 fatty acid which is more stable than either the n-3 or n-6 PUFA. However, we only benefit from the anti-inflammatory properties of this n-9 fatty acid if quantities of the other PUFAs are kept in check. When PUFA consumption is excessive, the very enzyme systems which elongate and desaturate Oleic Acid to make Mead Acid are suppressed. Yet, ironically enough, the *presence* of Mead Acid is an indication of an essential fatty acid *"deficiency"* in the body. Lord help our ass-backwards logic....

Estrogen—there's a lot of misinformation surrounding this hormone. For instance, it's often referred to as the female hormone. But males produce it, too. In fact, estrogen is what begins the masculinization of the male fetus in utero. So differentiating it from other hormones the body makes by implying it's unique to a specific gender is simply incorrect. Another example is its wide use in hormone replacement treatment (HRT), at least until studies such as the *2003 Women's Health Initiative* revealed some alarming side effects of supplemental estrogen. Estrogen increases prolactin which accelerates bone loss. It augments the level of serotonin in the body—and that shouldn't make anyone happy. It stimulates parathyroid hormone and cortisol. Blood clots, heart disease, and even the incidence of some cancers were all shown to increase with supplementation. Still, the practice of prescribing estrogen to ameliorate the symptoms of everything from PMS to menopause remains as common as it is misguided.

There are several actions by which estrogen severely impacts health—most notably by compromising energy production and setting the Seesaw of Sickness in motion. For starters, it blocks the activity of cytochrome oxidase. Without this critical respiratory enzyme, mitochondrial functioning is impaired. The mitochondria are the powerhouses of the cells. Thus, deficiencies here result in an immediate decline in ATP production. As Douglas Wallace of the National Academy of Sciences states:

Medicine fails to solve many of today's common, complex diseases, because the fundamental paradigm is wrong: the medical establishment has spent far too long focusing on anatomy and ignoring energy—specifically, mitochondria.

Estrogen lowers CO_2 generation, too, thereby inhibiting the delivery of oxygen. Indeed, tissue hypoxia is one of the detrimental effects estrogen produces when allowed to accumulate beyond normal levels. It also wastes vitamin B_6, which is intimately involved in glucose metabolism. To top it all off, excess estrogen adversely impacts the thyroid via at least three different ways: increasing thyroid binding globulin, interfering with the conversion of T_4 to T_3, and blocking the uptake of thyroid hormone.

Estrogen's influence on health is magnified secondary to its deleterious effect on albumin which is lowered when estrogen is excessive. Without adequate levels of albumin to bind various dangerous substances until the liver is ready to deal with them, detoxification is hampered and the onslaught of toxins begins to build up. And, ironically, estrogen makes the Kupffer cells of the liver actually more sensitive to endotoxin—15 times more sensitive according to one study. An excerpt from *Hepatology Elsewhere* noted:

> *...estrogens enhance the toxicity of endotoxin in vivo by at least three independent mechanisms. First, estrogens reduce serum lipoproteins, thereby impairing an important pathway for endotoxin neutralization. Second, estrogens increase CD14 expression on macrophages, which increases the capacity for these cells to bind endotoxin and produce cytokines and reactive oxygen intermediates. Estrogens also increase synthesis of LBP; this could have positive or negative effects on endotoxin toxicity because LBP facilitates LPS trafficking to both signaling (toxic) and nonsignaling (neutralizing) pathways. However, in the context of the two previous alterations, which tip the balance in favor of signaling pathways, LBP would serve to amplify LPS sampling even further.*

As endotoxin levels increase, liver function, of course, decreases. The result is energy production eventually declines, too. Then detoxification slows down even more. Estrogen is cleared no where near as efficiently as it should be, and the whole cycle perpetuates a condition known as estrogen dominance.

Compared to their male counterparts, women have a head start on reaching the precarious state of estrogen dominance. Men, however, are quickly closing the gap by following questionable nutrition and lifestyle principles. Of course, maybe that's one competition you're not overly concerned with as a man. That's actually okay— maybe even prudent. See, *stress* is a prime stimulator of aromatase—the enzyme which converts testosterone to estrogen in males. So one of the best strategies a guy can use to keep from developing moobies is to simply not worry about it. But it might also help if he minimized inflammation and polyunsaturated fatty acids as both of these are major players in the induction and activation of this particular enzyme, too.

Another way to keep estrogen within physiological norms is to avoid the sources of xenoestrogens commonly encountered in modern living. Xenoestrogens are synthetic or even naturally occurring chemical compounds that mimic the effects of endogenous estrogen. My readers may recognize Bisphenol A as one of the toxins found in plastic or cans. You may also realize that estrogenic substances are often used by plants as chemical defenses against the animals which prey upon them. Yet, in an effort at full disclosure, I have opted to include a more detailed list for the reader to become familiar with below:

Common Xenoestrogens

- **4-Methylbenzylidene camphor or 4-MBC** (sunscreens)
- **Alkylphenol** (detergents, fuels, and lubricants)
- **Atrazine** (weed killer)
- **Benzophenones** (sunscreens)
- **Butylated hydroxyanisole or BHA** (preservative)
- **Bisphenol A or BPA** (found in plastics and cans)
- **Chlorine** (in drinking water—refer to the Hydration section of *Spot On*)
- **Commercially raised meats and animal products**
- **Conventionally grown produce**
- **DDT** (insecticide banned in the USA but sold to other countries for use in agriculture and then brought back for sale here)
- **DEHP** (plasticizer for PVC)
- **Dieldrin** (insecticide)
- **Dioxin** (byproduct of the chlorine industry)
- **Endosulfan** (insecticide)
- **Erythrosine / FD&C Red No. 3**
- **Ethinylestradiol** (combined oral contraceptive pill)
- **Flax**
- **Heptachlor** (insecticide)
- **Lavender Oil** (skincare and cleaning)
- **Metalloestrogens** (a class of inorganic xenoestrogens)
- **Methoxychlor** (insecticide)
- **Nonylphenol** (industrial surfactants, laboratory detergents, and pesticides)
- **Parabens** (methylparaben, ethylparaben, propylparaben, and butylparaben—all commonly used as preservatives in personal care products)
- **Polychlorinated biphenyls or PCBs** (adhesives, electrical oils, lubricants, and paints)
- **Pentachlorophenol** (general biocide and wood preservative)
- **Phenosulfothiazine** (type of red dye)
- **Phenoxyethanol** (skincare products)
- **Phthalates** (plasticizers)
- **Placental Extract** (shampoos and skincare products)
- **Propyl gallate (**cosmetics, hair products, adhesives, and lubricants)
- **PUFAS** (of course)
- **Soy**
- **Tea Tree Oil** (skincare and cleaning products)

The previous list is by no means exhaustive. From the pesticide industry to the manufacturers of personal care products, you're being exposed to various sources of estrogens from all sides. And, despite what you may think, I'm truly not trying to be an alarmist. I just want you well informed. Ignorance may be bliss, but it's still ignorance. And it's the type of ignorance which can cost you your health. My hope with this little lesson is it allows you to be more cognizant of what you put in your body and what you put *on* your body as well. Because there's one final injustice which an excessive accumulation of estrogen can cause. Activating an enzyme called transglutaminase, estrogen makes some cells more sensitive to gluten. So, if a little education helps you learn how to minimize estrogen through sound nutrition/lifestyle principles, you can quite literally have your cake and eat it, too.

Barbara Seaman's *The Greatest Experiment Ever Performed on Women: Exploding the Estrogen Myth* is an excellent resource for my readers who would like to explore this subject in greater detail.

Fructose—thanks to high fructose corn syrup (HFCS), fructose has a bad rap. Yet, if you'll recall from Chapter Six of this section, it's actually quite low on the Glycemic Index. What's more important to consider, however, is the unique ability of fructose to be used as fuel in the presence of polyunsaturated fatty acids. Normally, PUFAs inhibit the oxidation of sugar for fuel. So foods such as bread or even rice—polysaccharides made up of chains of glucose molecules—are not efficiently utilized and can readily cause blood sugar handling issues or other potential health problems. This effect is avoided when fructose is consumed. So, there's more to this simple sugar than most diet gurus would have you believe.

Medium Chain Triglyceride (MCT)—an ongoing theme in this book has been the importance of the middle road in maintaining health. Thus, it should come as no surprise that medium chain triglycerides are some of the most beneficial fats to include in one's diet. Unlike longer chain fatty acids, MCTs do not require bile to be broken down nor do they require the carnitine transport system to enter the mitochondria. The unique characteristics of these fats allow them be readily used as fuel rather than being stored in the body's adipose tissue. Indeed, farmers looking for an inexpensive way to fatten their livestock discovered this fact for themselves when animals fed coconut oil—an MCT—actually lost weight. Guess they let their subscription to the *Journal of Lipid Research* expire. Otherwise they may have read studies which concluded:

> ...diets rich in medium-chain fatty acids (MCFAs) have been associated with increased oxidative metabolism and reduced adiposity, with few deleterious effects on insulin action....MCFA-fed mice exhibited increased energy expenditure, reduced adiposity, and better glucose tolerance compared with LCFA-fed mice.

Coconut oil, specifically, has a number of qualities which make it beneficial for human health beyond its metabolic effect. It protects the heart from cardiovascular disease:

its [coconut oil's] cardioprotective effects may make this a possible dietary intervention in isolation or in combination with exercise to help reduce the burden of CVDs.

It also shows strong antifungal effects:

It is noteworthy that coconut oil was active against species of Candida at 100% concentration compared to fluconazole. Coconut oil should be used in the treatment of fungal infections in view of emerging drug-resistant Candida species.

The predominate fatty acid found in coconuts—lauric acid—is also touted for its antibacterial properties:

The obtained data highlight the potential of using lauric acid as an alternative treatment for antibiotic therapy of acne vulgaris.

As well as its antiviral potential:

...it can be concluded that lauric acid inhibited a late maturation stage in the replicative cycle of JUNV [Junin virus].

A medium chain triglyceride, lauric acid's antifungal, antibacterial, and antiviral properties have been known for years. I mentioned its use in the treatment of AIDS earlier in this section. Specifically, it is converted in the body into monolaurin which acts on lipid-coated viruses (like HIV, herpes, and others) and destroys them. But I've also come across studies demonstrating the benefits of coconut oil in the treatment of osteoporosis (http://www.ncbi.nlm.nih.gov/pubmed/23024690) as well as in the treatment of arthritis (http://www.ncbi.nlm.nih.gov/pubmed/24613207?dopt=Abstract). I've even seen research discussing how virgin coconut oil protects the liver from acetaminophen (http://www.hindawi.com/journals/ecam/2011/142739/).

Whether coconut oil can benefit neurological conditions such as Alzheimer's has sparked a heated debate recently. There's plenty of evidence to support that premise, so it wouldn't surprise me if most of the naysayers have some sort of allegiance to the pharmaceutical industry. Consider, for instance, the abstract of a study below:

Glucose is the brain's principal energy substrate. In Alzheimer's disease (AD), there appears to be a pathological decrease in the brain's ability to use glucose. Neurobiological evidence suggests that ketone bodies are an effective alternative energy substrate for the brain. Elevation of plasma ketone body levels through an oral dose of medium chain triglycerides (MCTs) may improve cognitive functioning in older adults with memory disorders. On separate days, 20 subjects with AD or mild cognitive impairment consumed a drink containing emulsified MCTs or placebo. Significant increases in levels of the ketone body *beta-hydroxybutyrate (beta-OHB) were observed 90 min after treatment (P=0.007) when cognitive tests were administered. beta-OHB elevations were moderated by apolipoprotein E (APOE) genotype (P=0.036). For 4+ subjects, beta-OHB levels continued to rise between the 90 and 120 min blood draws in the treatment condition, while the beta-OHB levels of 4- subjects held constant (P<0.009). On cognitive testing, MCT treatment facilitated performance on the Alzheimer's Disease Assessment Scale-Cognitive Subscale (ADAS-cog) for 4- subjects, but not for 4+ subjects (P=0.04). Higher ketone values were associated with greater improvement in paragraph recall with MCT treatment relative to placebo across all subjects (P=0.02). Additional research is warranted to determine the therapeutic benefits of MCTs for patients with AD and how APOE-4 status may mediate beta-OHB efficacy.*

Or this one:

Ketogenic compounds derived from medium chain triglyceride (MCT) oils have been claimed to have beneficial health effects in the Alzheimer's disease (AD] mainly attributed to its medium chain triglycerides. AD is known to have been characterized by early and region specific decline in cerebral glucose metabolism. It is hypothesized that Alzheimer brain tends to preferentially utilize ketones generated from medium chain triglycerides in light of decreased glucose metabolism to improve cognition. Extra virgin coconut oil with predominance of MCT content was used in subjects with moderate to severe AD to examine its efficacy in improving cognitive performance. Methods: Daily oral administration of extra virgin coconut oil (20 gm) was evaluated in 31 subjects with predominantly moderate to severe AD diagnosed as per DSM IV TR criteria for AD in a 6 week trial using quasi experimental non randomized pre-post intervention design. Subjects were on a normal diet and continued taking approved AD medications. Primary cognitive end points were mean change from baseline in the AD Assessment Scale-Cognitive subscale [ADAS-Cog], and Clinicians Interview based Impression of Change Plus Caregivers input [CIBIC-Plus]. Active oil administration continued for 4 weeks from baseline with successive ratings on measures of cognitive change at 2, 4 and 6 weeks respectively. Results: There was a significant difference between the ADAS-Cog scores from baseline over repeated ratings at 2, 4 and 6 weeks (Mauchly's Chi Square $X2 = 61.1$, $\varepsilon=0.4$, $F =14$, $p=0.00$, $\eta2=0.31$). Post hoc comparisons of ADAS-Cog scores from baseline at 4 and 6 weeks were similar [At 4 weeks, Mean difference=4.1, P=0.00, C.I= (1.4-6.7); at 6 weeks, Mean difference=4.1, p=0.00, C.I= (1.0-7.2). The response rate of CIBIC-Plus defined as improved or no change was significantly improved over successive ratings from 2 weeks to 6 weeks (Cochran's Q=22.5, df=2, P=.00). No statistically significant difference could be noted for the total cholesterol, Triglycerides and LDL fractions over the study trial except for the HDL fraction over repeated measures at 4 and 6 weeks over baseline (Mauchly's Chi Square $X2$ (df=2)=6.5, $\varepsilon=0.8$, F (df 1.6, 49.9)=6.4, p=0.005, $_n2=0.17$). Conclusions: Addition of adjunctive coconut oil is likely to have beneficial effects in cognitive performance for those suffering

98

from moderate to severe AD and the effects were sustained for at least 2 weeks after the oil administration stopped. No deleterious effects on the overall lipid profile could be elicited.

After three concussions, I want to do anything I can to decrease my chances of developing Alzheimer's. And though I guess I could do crossword puzzles, making smoothies everyday is less time consuming. Thus, I put at least a tablespoon or two of coconut oil in each one—for all those health reasons cited above and more. In fact, one of the most important benefits of consuming coconut oil daily could be that it helps offset the amount of PUFAs in the diet, thereby minimizing the toxic effects of these fats. Many open-minded experts agree, with some now recommending 20-25 grams of lauric acid a day. However, there is no current RDA for this nutrient. Then again, how could there be? The best sources are breast milk and coconuts. The former you can't sell in stores. And the latter, of course, is too high in saturated fat— still evil in the eyes of the USDA. Of course, in light of the health of most Americans, that vision is somewhat suspect....

Melatonin—a derivative of serotonin, this hormone made from tryptophan in the pineal gland is another misunderstood and, thus, often abused substance. As Ray Peat states:

Many health foods stores are now selling melatonin, to induce sleep and "prevent cancer." They have taken some information out of context, and don't realize how dangerous melatonin is. It makes the brain sluggish, causes sex organs to shrink, and damages immunity by shrinking the thymus gland. It suppresses thyroid and progesterone, and increases estrogen. It is the hormone of darkness and winter, and is produced in the pineal gland by any stress which increases adrenalin.

Thankfully, it's inhibited by bright light (see *Light Therapy* below). Yet, if for some reason you still think you should supplement with it, may I suggest you sleep on that?

Parathyroid Hormone (PTH)—as its name would suggest, PTH is a hormone secreted by the chief cells of the parathyroid gland in response to low levels of calcium in the blood (or a poor calcium to phosphorus ratio). It's also stimulated by adrenaline. Thus, it could easily be considered a "*stress*" hormone. The primary action of PTH is to increase blood calcium levels, but it does so by stealing from the main calcium reservoirs of the body—the bones and teeth. Some of this leached calcium can overflow into the soft tissue of the body, resulting in various pathologies. While those looking on the bright side might point out that PTH helps convert vitamin D to its active form, thereby enhancing calcium absorption, the dark side of this hormone finds it strongly associated with high blood pressure, inflammation, and even tumor growth.

Progesterone—progesterone is synthesized from Pregnenolone, which in turn is derived from cholesterol. Like cholesterol, a high concentration of it can be found in the brain, alluding to its many protective qualities outside of its role in supporting pregnancy. Most important of these, perhaps, is its opposition of estrogen. Via action on the protein estrogen receptor as well as the enzyme responsible for stimulating estrogen production, progesterone keeps its counterpart in check. One could say it's the *good cop* to estrogen's *bad cop*. In fact, so-called estrogen dominance can easily be a case of progesterone deficiency when this hormone is not produced in sufficient quantities to lower estrogen to non-toxic levels.

Progesterone also inactivates tryptophan hydroxylase. This is the enzyme responsible for sending tryptophan down the serotonin pathway—a route best left less traveled as you'll learn by referring to the section on *Serotonin* below. Other benefits of progesterone include improved functioning of the mitochondria and decreased lipid peroxidation. It also relaxes smooth muscles (enhancing respiration and circulation) and increases core temperature. Progesterone has anti-inflammatory properties and strengthens the immune system, too, reportedly by rejuvenating the thymus. Finally (though I could go on), it helps to maintain blood sugar which is why Ray Peat writes *"progesterone is probably the most perfect antiestrogenic hormone, and therefore an anti-stress and anti-aging hormone...."*

Pregnenolone—shown to improve memory, boost mood, and fight stress, this is the mother of all hormones—literally. Pregnenolone is the hormone from which all the other steroid hormones are made. However, this production follows a specific hierarchy as dictated by the body's need to survive:

1. Stress hormones
2. Repair hormones
3. Sex hormones

Think about it. If your life is in danger, would you really need a huge surge of testosterone to quickly grow hair on your chest and lower your voice? Yeah, I might think twice about messing with you if you suddenly transformed into the Barry White version of Sasquatch. But many threats we faced during the course of human evolution probably weren't intimidated so easily. In most of those cases, we either had to fight or run for our lives. And that meant stress hormone production. A more detailed explanation of this critical process can be found in the following illustration:

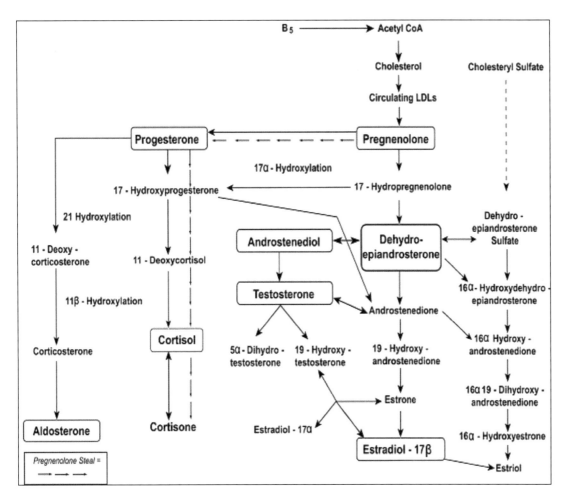

Now, draw you attention to the dotted arrows running horizontally from Pregnenolone to Progesterone at the top center of the diagram. They illustrate what is termed *Pregnenolone Steal.* To put it simply, when the demand for stress hormones (which are produced preferentially over the other steroid hormones) is chronic, the body converts most of the raw material—pregnenolone—into cortisol. Repair and sex hormone production slows down as fewer building blocks for their synthesis are available. Conventional thinking makes this whole scenario even worse. For if pregnenolone is the mother, then cholesterol would have to be the grandmother. Yet the big bad wolf of modern medicine pretty much did away with her. Thus, without her matriarchal contribution, health has quickly become the stuff of fairy tales.

Proteolytic Enzymes—various digestive enzymes, such as bromelain or papain, can be good pain relievers and a healthy alternative to Non-Steroidal Anti-inflammatory Drugs (NSAIDs). Studies show NSAIDs actually delay the healing process. Additionally the damage to the liver as well as various organs involved in digestion warrant caution when using over-the-counter or prescription forms of these drugs. Proteolytic enzymes work as natural anti-inflammatories when taken on an empty stomach. Normally present in certain foods (bromelain is extracted from pineapple, for example), these enzymes help break down proteins in your gut, improving digestion and assimilation. However, when taken away from meals, these same substances break down excess fibrin in your circulatory system and in other connective tissue (e.g., muscle) which often deprive the tissue of the essential blood necessary for healing (via oxygen delivery and the removal of metabolic waste).

Serotonin—it makes me sad how people constantly refer to serotonin as the *"happy"* hormone. There's probably a drug for that—actually, I'm sure there is...but I think I'll pass. The evidence behind these anti-depressants is sketchy at best, and shady is likely a more accurate qualifier. After all, there's a boat load of money to be made. And when the only thing shakier than the foundation of the depression theory is the evidence behind the efficacy of the product which *"treats"* said depression, certain miraculous leaps are bound to be made.

> *Many patients are led to believe, by their physicians and by advertising, that antidepressant drugs will act on the biological cause of their depressed state by rectifying a "chemical imbalance"....our analysis indicates that there are no specific antidepressant drugs, that most of the short-term effects of antidepressants are shared by many other drugs, and that long-term drug treatment with antidepressants or any other drugs has not been shown to lead to long-term elevation of mood. We suggest that the term "antidepressant" should be abandoned.*
> (excerpted from http://www.ncbi.nlm.nih.gov/pmc/articles/PMC1472553/)

Serotonin reuptake inhibitors (SSRIs) specifically, are proposed to *"work"* by increasing the action of serotonin in the brain. This theory would make sense if the etiology of depression were simply a reduction in the body's levels of this neurotransmitter; or even if the actions of serotonin were as well understood as the pharmaceutical companies would have you believe. However, a lot of research casts serious doubt on both of those ideas. For example, a study involving mice which had been genetically depleted of serotonin showed they did not display increased levels of depression. The authors concluded that the behavior of the mice *"questions the role of 5HT in depression."* Indeed, when consideration is given to some of the recognized biological actions of serotonin, the view that more of it must be better quickly falls apart.

Approximately 95% of serotonin is synthesized in the intestines by the enterochromaffin cells where its primary action is to trigger peristalsis. And while an increase in intestinal contractions is a benefit when the body needs to expel a poison or otherwise noxious substance, excessive stimulation comes at a cost. In this way, the production of serotonin is much like activation of the Sympathetic Nervous System. Cortisol and adrenaline can be lifesaving under the right circumstances. Chronic stimulation of these stress hormones, however, can literally kill you. Indeed, there are very few biological processes where a consistent state of excess doesn't eventually result in serious consequences to the health of the human body. More is most definitely not always better.

Unfortunately, anything which irritates the gut wall (e.g., cellulose) increases the production of serotonin. And it is this synthesis of serotonin which is of particular interest in light of a 2014 article which appeared in *Nature Medicine*. The paper's authors discovered that suppression of the so-called happy hormone actually produced an effect which should make some folks downright giddy.

> *We find that Tph1-deficient mice fed a high-fat diet (HFD) are protected from obesity, insulin resistance and nonalcoholic fatty liver disease (NAFLD) while exhibiting greater energy expenditure by BAT. Small-molecule chemical inhibition of Tph1 in HFD-fed mice mimics the benefits ascribed to Tph1 genetic deletion, effects that depend on UCP1-mediated thermogenesis. The inhibitory effects of serotonin on energy expenditure are cell autonomous, as serotonin blunts ß-adrenergic induction of the thermogenic program in brown and beige adipocytes in vitro. As obesity increases peripheral serotonin, the inhibition of serotonin signaling or its synthesis in adipose tissue may be an effective treatment for obesity and its comorbidities.*

Or to put those findings in plain English, I'll quote one of the study's co-authors who said, *"Our results are quite striking and indicate that inhibiting the production of this hormone may be very effective for reversing obesity and related metabolic diseases including diabetes."*

The above research focused primarily on what's termed brown adipose tissue and how its thermogenic potential is blunted by peripheral serotonin. Yet, there are likely other factors involved here, too. For instance, serotonin is known to exacerbate hypoglycemia which, in turn, limits the conversion of thyroxine (T_4) into the more biologically active thyroid hormone triiodothyronine (T_3). More metabolic damage is done via a serotonin-induced decrease in brain ATP which then activates anaerobic glycolysis. The resulting lactic acid interferes with mitochondrial respiration by opposing the production of CO_2. Additionally, the concomitant increase in ACTH with serotonin contributes to the rise in cortisol which triggers tryptophan to be released secondary to muscle catabolism. More tryptophan means more building blocks for the synthesis of serotonin, perpetuating this cycle of stress and its adverse impact on metabolism.

And the Seesaw of Sickness keeps on going...

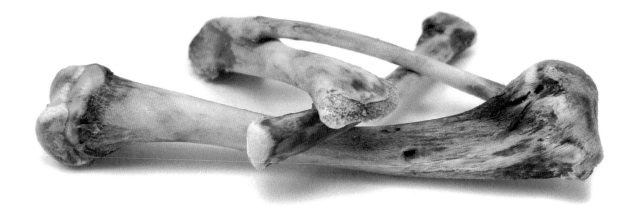

It's not leftovers that are wasteful, but those who either don't know what to do with them or can't be bothered.

—Julian Baggini

I don't expect you to assimilate everything. Most of us learn best in layers, so I urge you not to be discouraged if some of the concepts you've just been fed are too big for you to swallow right now. That's to be expected. Hell, if there was nothing in this section you really had to chew over and think about, you'd probably be disappointed. At the very least, I know you'd be unsatisfied.

I remember when I first started studying the work of my mentor, Paul Chek. I had just dropped a load of cash on his correspondence course entitled *Scientific Back Conditioning*. My ideas of how to train the human body had been honed by some of the best cycling coaches in the world, and I thought my anatomy knowledge was pretty good, too. Yet, when I listened to Paul's first lecture, it seemed like he was speaking in a different language. Literally every fifth word I could hardly pronounce, much less understand. And as I sat watching the VHS tape of him speaking (yes, it was a long time ago...), I thought to myself that I may have wasted my money.

An investment in self, as I would eventually learn, always yields the best returns. So every time I finished a lecture, I *rewound* the tape to play it again (I probably would've cut my learning time in half if I could've simply pushed a button and skipped back to the start). Most of those sessions had me cycling on the indoor trainer or running on the treadmill. Coupling movement with learning always worked well for me. And each time I gleaned a little bit more. I remember learning from someone—I bet it was Paul—that you have to read and/or hear something seven times before you fully comprehend it. For some subjects it's probably more. For some it may be less. All I know is I watched each of those tapes so many times I could probably still quote some of the dialogue. Part of me would love to test that theory, but I don't have a VCR anymore.

Yet it's not just memorization. Any piece of insight you may have gained from reading this section is no better than the decades of misinformation we've all been poisoned with until you actually apply it. Don't stuff yourself in one sitting. Don't force it all down just so you can easily spit it back out. Likewise, don't rush to share anything in these pages until you've truly tasted each bite—until you can describe the nuances of every fact in flavorful detail. Knowledge is a nutrient which you have to feed yourself first before you can really nourish others.

A word of caution here. Just as the macronutrients work together to bring out the nutrition in a particular food, so, too, any combination of facts can affect different people in various ways. Some may suffer paralysis from analysis—you just don't know how to proceed. A mental constipation of sorts, this is a sign that you've taken in much more information than you're capable of using at your present level of understanding. If that's the case, I suggest focusing on one chapter at a time. You can even break that chapter down into smaller bite size pieces, picking a concept which appears ripe or appealing to you in some way. Savor it until you own it and don't move on until you're ready for another helping.

Along with indecision, a taste of truth can trigger other reactions as well. I wouldn't be surprised if some of you were angry. After all, you've been led astray. We're so far removed now from how we were designed to eat, that health is getting harder and harder to recognize. Stats from the Center for Disease Control show that 34.9% of the United States is obese—a full 78.9 million Americans. Unfortunately, other industrialized countries are giving us a good run for our money (or at least a slow waddle). Heart disease kills over 600,000 people a year in this country. Diabetes affects another 30 million. And if you don't know someone with cancer these days, I suggest you get out more.

Some of you may actually fear food now. That was never my intention, of course, so I hope it's not many of my readers. But if the food you eat is frightening, maybe you should be scared of it. To me it's like automobiles. Cars don't need to be feared. But you do have to handle them with respect. Yet respect rarely shares the plate of the food we eat today. Most of us don't even know where that food comes from. In interviews with children, Jamie Oliver found that fewer than half of the kids he polled could recognize most common farm animals. You have to learn how to drive before you are safe behind the wheel. Likewise, learning how and what to eat is the only way we won't end up digging our own graves with a knife and fork.

What's sad is that people who are actually conscious of what they eat have recently been labeled as having a disorder. *Orthoexia Nervosa* is not an official term in the *DSM-IV* (the Diagnostic and Statistical Manual used by mental health practitioners to diagnosis mental health problems), but it is quickly becoming a widely accepted diagnosis in the mental health community. That absolutely boggles my mind! Look—I know people have all types of hang ups with foods. Serious conditions such as anorexia or bulimia or even body dysmorphia are real problem from which many people suffer. Yet, in my professional experience, I've come to realize your consciousness of health reflects the health of your consciousness. If people want to label me in the hopes I'm gonna ask my doctor "if Drug X is right for" me, then go ahead. Maybe I just need to go to Asparagus Anonymous meetings....

Others of you, unfortunately, may actually feel guilty after reading this section. That's the last thing I want, but I understand your reaction. Most of you have done your damndest to teach your children the importance of nutrition. You studiously follow the guidelines the government seems to revise each year only to realize that the dietary education you've been giving your children is really nothing more than an expert lesson in how to be sick.

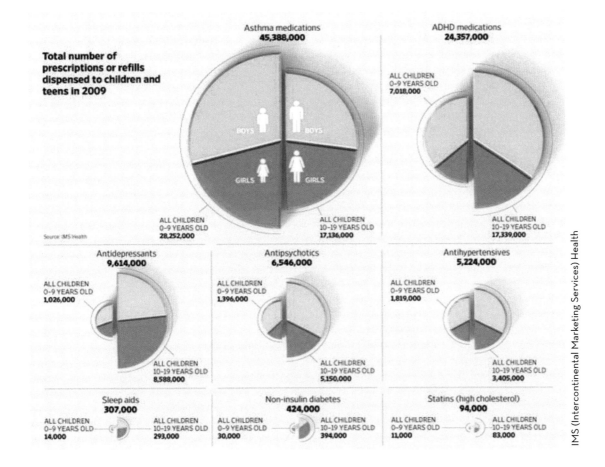

IMS (Intercontinental Marketing Services) Health

Looking at those stats above, I'd say our kids have been excellent students. So good, in fact, that they have the dubious honor of being the first generation of Americans born who won't live as long as their parents. A 2010 report by the CDC shows that life expectancy dropped for the first time in this country. Specifically, increases in Alzheimer's, high blood pressure, kidney disease, suicide, and flu/pneumonia were to blame. Yet all of these conditions are strongly influenced in one way or another by nutrition.

"Yeah, but when I was young, I could eat whatever I wanted."

Really? And what does that prove? People *love* using age as excuse. The number I usually hear thrown around is forty: *"When you turn forty, your metabolism slows down"* or *"In your forties, your body just begins to change."* Of course, many of the people making these kinds of statements are walking billboards for their own claims. Science would be quick to point that N=1 in this case. An effective rebuttal might ask science to simply consider the majority of our population. Heck, just 30 minutes of television is enough to convince most of us that with age comes high cholesterol, low sex drive, and midsection weight gain.

That, of course, is part of the problem. The thirty minutes of TV when we're ten is one hour when we're twenty. Those two drinks a night at twenty are four drinks a night at forty. Each injustice our young bodies endured in youth is magnified with each passing year until...

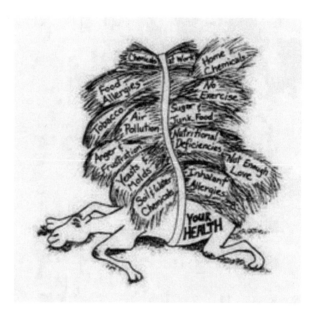

You may think that all your unhealthy habits didn't impact you when you were younger. But here's the truth. The Froot Loops you ate as a kid (or last week for some of you reading this)—that box of cereal was still void of nutrition back then. The cost for your body to digest and assimilate it as a child was no less expensive than it is now. You weren't impervious to processed food or caloric excess. That you didn't get sick or fat eating junk food every day had nothing to do with how old you were so much as how many years of doing this shit you now have under your belt.

You're really only as old as your habits.

The study of Epigenetics explains one of the reasons why life expectancy is decreasing for the first time in recorded history. Basically, our DNA stores memory. So any choice we made which led to suboptimal health when we were younger has even more and greater adverse consequences on our children. When researchers feed rats a typical American diet, subsequent generations express significant increases in body fat. In essence, scientists have discovered that the food we eat today will impact the health of our grandchildren.

Another example is a book entitled *Pottenger's Cats*. Though written way back in the 1940s, it does an eerily accurate job of describing exactly how our nutritional past is still a part of our present. Dr. Pottenger compared the effects of raw versus processed foods in experiments which he conducted over the course of ten years. As carnivores, the cats Pottenger fed a traditional diet of raw meat and raw milk thrived. But the cats fed on cooked or otherwise processed foods, in contrast, suffered a variety of disorders—from physical degeneration to changes in personality, becoming increasingly aggressive and violent. Parasite infestation, hypothyroidism, and other disorders affected the cats as early as the first generation. And by the third and fourth generations, their ability to procreate was severely limited.

Now, there are definitely more than a few criticisms of Pottenger's work. One being obvious—we're not cats. That's true. However, people my age *are* the third generation of processed food eaters. And it's freaking scary when you consider the number of people of my generation who are unable to get pregnant—not to mention the amount of money spent on Viagra and Cialis each year! No, we're not cats. Yet for the past seventy-five to one hundred years humans have been part of a disastrous experiment, eating foods and ingesting chemicals that have never before been a part of our evolutionary history. The modern diet is exposing our genetic weaknesses which we are simply spoon feeding our children with every bite we take.

Ignorance gets passed down, too—though I don't think that can be explained by Epigenetics. It's simply that we've all become so accustomed to feeling like crap that we have no idea what health feels like anymore. We're so sick and tired that we don't even recognize when our lifestyle choices make us feel sick and tired. It's like having a clean glass of water and a dirty glass of water. Put a sprinkle of dirt in the pure one, and you'll taste it right away. But add some to the dirty one, and you'll continue drinking because you don't even notice it.

We need to raise our baseline of health because right now it's deep in the toilet. You know the health of your country has gone to crap when we have "*awareness*" months for various diseases. Illness has become so easy it's hard to find someone who isn't sick! What is this teaching our children? What are the lessons they're learning?

One cannot know health by studying sickness.

It's said that when the first ships sailed over the Atlantic to the New World, the natives couldn't even see them. Something so strange was so incomprehensible to what they knew as reality their minds just couldn't register what their eyes were seeing. I want my son to be able to accept that health is possible. He should know that health is *real*, that it's his birthright. Like the great Shamans of old, his vision of what's possible should allow him greater clarity when he begins exploring his own infinite potential.

Here's daddy, Son.

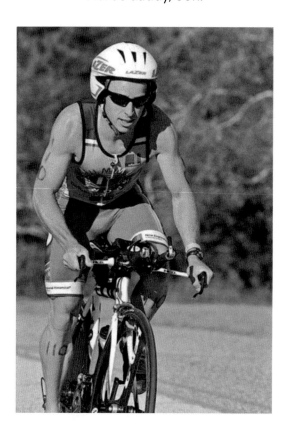

And you can be better than me....

Vit A
- egg yolks
- liver
- milk/cheese

Essential to cellular metabolism, Vitamin A is a fat-soluble nutrient that aids in the production of pregnenolone, progesterone, and the other youth-associated steroids. A deficiency of vitamin A can slow down the conversion of cholesterol to these important hormones, creating what is, in effect, a state of estrogen dominance. While many people believe carrots and other plant sources are a good source of vitamin A, the nutrient found in these foods is actually beta carotene—the precursor to retinol which is the active form of this essential vitamin. PUFAs waste vitamin A, one of the many reasons these toxic oils should be minimized in the diet.

Vit B
- eggs
- liver
- milk

B_1 needs increase as carbohydrate increases. B_3 (niacinamide) helps lower free fatty acids (e.g., PUFAs), therefore being a good supplement for many. B_6 needs increase as protein increases. A deficiency of B vitamins, all of which are water-soluble, prevents the liver from efficiently eliminating estrogen.

Vit C
- fruit
- orange juice
- milk

The vitamin which put orange juice on the map—vitamin C (also known as ascorbic acid) is arguably the world's most familiar nutrient. A water-soluble vitamin with strong antioxidant properties, greater quantities of this nutrient are actually found in many other foods, including red pepper. Another misconception is that vitamin C helps prevent the common cold. Studies do not support this belief, though a modest effect on the duration of colds has been consistently observed. However, it does work pretty well for the synthesis of collagen—one of the benefits sailors suffering from scurvy during long voyages would have appreciated. It also is involved in protein metabolism, the synthesis of neurotransmitters, and research shows it may play a role in fat oxidation as well.

NOTE: Vitamin C facilitates the absorption of iron. Thus, for those with issues of iron toxicity, consuming foods rich in ascorbic acid is best avoided when consuming high-iron foods.

Vit D

- butter
- eggs
- fish
- liver
- sun (the best source as D_3 produced via sun exposure is self limiting due to an exquisite biofeedback mechanism)

D_3 is intimately involved in keeping us healthy, thus it's commonly referred to as the immunity vitamin. But that's not physiologically accurate; it's actually a secosteroid in the same family as all the other steroid hormones. Cholecalciferol, or Vitamin D_3, aids in calcium absorption while down regulating the production of parathyroid hormone. A study published in the journal *Nature Immunology* details how vitamin D protects the body by activating T cells—an integral part of the immune system:

> *When a T cell is exposed to a foreign pathogen, it extends a signaling device or 'antenna' known as a vitamin D receptor, with which it searches for vitamin D. This means the T cell must have vitamin D or activation of the cell will cease. If the T cells cannot find enough vitamin D in the blood, they won't even begin to mobilize.*

This finding may help explain why "flu/cold season" occurs predominately during the winter months: http://triumphtraining.com/blogs/blog/6364690-the-answer-vitamin-d-deficiency

NOTE: Increasing vitamin D intake without adding vitamin K increases the potential for calcium deposits in the arterial walls, reducing their elasticity. The Vit D_3/K_2 supplement I recommend can be found on my website (see the Resources section below).

Vit E

- liver
- milk
- olive oil

Essential for the absorption of vitamin A, Vitamin E is a well known antioxidant. This fat-soluble vitamin possesses anti-estrogenic properties (thus, making it pro-thyroid), and helps protect against lipid peroxidation as well as iron toxicity. Vitamin E has also been shown to improve the oxygenation of the body's cells and can be applied topically to aid in the healing of scars.

Vit K

- butter (grass-fed sources)
- hard cheeses
- kiwi (not a great fruit choice for many)
- mineral broth
- organ meats

Vitamin K$_2$ helps keep calcium where it should be—in the bones and teeth instead of in the soft tissues of the body where it contributes to disease and dysfunction. Studies show it effective against prostate cancer. K$_2$ also possesses antioxidant properties, helps down regulate parathyroid hormone, and helps normalize the viscosity of the blood. Bacteria in the small intestines will convert Vitamin K to K$_2$, but only if the gut remains healthy. Thus, antibiotics or foods not suitable for human digestion can inhibit this conversion.

Calcium
- dairy
- bone broths (use a vinegar to leach the minerals from the bone into the broth)
- egg shells (see the egg shell recipe in the Resources section)

Sufficient quantities of calcium keep parathyroid hormone low while also increasing the likelihood of tryptophan converting to niacin rather than serotonin. An important mineral for cellular communication, calcium is involved in muscle contraction and is a key component in the electrical conduction system of the heart.

Copper
- cocoa
- liver
- low-fat fish
- shellfish

Found predominately in the brain, the liver, and the muscles of the body, copper has a number of important functions. It helps convert inactive thyroid hormone to the active form. It is also involved in the formation of red blood cells. A component of cytochrome oxidase—the enzyme essential for red light absorption—copper's role in optimal cellular respiration is arguably one of its key functions. A deficiency of copper can cause the body to retain excess iron which can be toxic in large amounts and damage iron-storing organs like the liver.

Magnesium
- bone broth
- coffee
- dark chocolate
- Epsom salt baths
- fruit
- magnesium carbonate, magnesium glycinate, etc
- meat

With 3751 magnesium binding sites identified in the human body, this mineral is gaining an increased level of respect among health practitioners. It keeps oxalates soluble, thereby preventing the formation of kidney stones. It reduces both aldosterone as well as ACTH levels in the body. Phase 2 detoxification in the liver (glucoronidation) requires magnesium to eliminate xenobiotics. The activity of HMG Co-A reductase—the enzyme which triggers cholesterol production in the liver—is predicated on magnesium, so a deficiency of this mineral can cause elevated levels of cholesterol on a lipid panel. And it's extraordinarily common to be deficient in magnesium—

especially in the hypothyroid, in whom it's one of the first minerals to be depleted. A final fact: magnesium is found in well over 300 enzymes including the ones involved in the synthesis and utilization of ATP. That means energy production. And in case you forgot about the Seesaw of Sickness, that means health.

Potassium
- bone broth
- coconut water
- fruit
- orange juice

Potassium accelerates the conversion of cholesterol to pregnenolone. An electrolyte, it has an intimate relationship with sodium. Its intake shows a positive association with bone density in elderly women, suggesting that increasing consumption of food rich in potassium may play a role in osteoporosis prevention. Got bananas?

Sodium
- Hains or Morton's Pickling Salt (with no anti-caking agents)
- Sea salt (males or women who are no longer menstruating may find that the mineral content, specifically iron, may cause levels in the body to become excessive)

Like sugar, salt is much maligned among health professionals. National dietary guidelines in the United States have long promoted an upper limit of 1500mg a day—a bit more than half a teaspoon—to protect against stroke and heart attacks. This *"protection"* comes in part from a small reduction in blood pressure when sodium intake is restricted. The issue of what constitutes normal blood pressure, however, has recently come under question (http://triumphtraining.com/blogs/blog/17298908-impact-of-diastolic-and-systolic-blood-pressure-on-mortality-implications-for-the-definition-of-normal).

Even if there is no consensus among health professionals regarding the definition of abnormal blood pressure, biochemistry takes a definite stance on the importance of sodium. Restriction increases level of adrenaline, cortisol, parathyroid hormone, prolactin, and serotonin. Additionally, insufficient sodium stimulates the synthesis of aldosterone in an effort to preserve salt (and water) in the body. Unfortunately, aldosterone causes both magnesium and potassium to be lost, the effect of which actually *increases* vasoconstriction and, therefore, blood pressure. Activation of the renin-angiotensin-aldosterone system (RAAS) has other impacts outside of its effect on blood pressure, too:

> *Emerging evidence supports a paradigm shift in our understanding of the renin-angiotensin-aldosterone system and in aldosterone's ability to promote insulin resistance and participate in the pathogenesis of the metabolic syndrome and resistant hypertension. Recent data suggest that excess circulating aldosterone promotes the development of both disorders by impairing insulin metabolic signaling and endothelial function, which in turn leads to insulin resistance and cardiovascular and renal structural and functional*

abnormalities. Indeed, hyperaldosteronism is associated with impaired pancreatic beta-cell function, skeletal muscle insulin sensitivity, and elevated production of proinflammatory adipokines from adipose tissue, which results in systemic inflammation and impaired glucose tolerance.

Sodium actually helps regulate blood sugar by aiding with absorption in the intestines. It also increases blood volume, which helps improve the delivery of nutrients to the cells. The effect is to restore energy production while at the same time reducing inflammation and helping to stabilize the cell. CO_2 production is enhanced; SNS activity is reduced; and thyroid function is improved. Indeed, instead of limiting sodium, my mentors have encouraged me to consume up to 3 teaspoons a day on food/in water. Ray Peat is one of the strongest advocates, stating:

...it is almost always unphysiological and irrational to restrict sodium intake, because reduced blood volume tends to reduce the deliver of oxygen and nutrients to all tissues, leading to many problems.

Even the mainstream finally appears to be addressing its pollution of misinformation as evidenced by the below comment from the Academy of Nutrition and Dietetics in 2015:

There is a distinct and growing lack of scientific consensus on making a single sodium consumption recommendation for all Americans, owing to a growing body of research suggesting that the low sodium intake levels recommended by the DGAC are actually associated with increased mortality for healthy individuals.

For more information on the importance of sodium in human physiology, refer to the Hydration section of *Spot On*.

Selenium
- egg yolks
- liver
- low-fat fish
- shellfish

Selenium is a powerful antioxidant involved in DNA synthesis and thyroid hormone metabolism. Studies indicate it may be preventive against certain types of cancers, most notably cancers of the prostate and bladder. Research also shows selenium is effective at reducing fluoride-induced damage to neurons. More details on the subject of fluoride toxicity are found in the Hydration section of *Spot On*.

Zinc
- beef
- lamb
- liver
- shellfish

Crucial for thyroid hormone metabolism, it should come as no surprise that zinc has a key role in immunity as well as wound healing. It also aids in vitamin A conversion and hydrochloric acid production while playing an important part in carbohydrate metabolism, too. An essential trace element contributing to the active center of approximately 300 different enzymes, zinc is essential for both taste and smell. Thus, when deficient, a person may have uncontrolled cravings as normal food intake is not sufficient for satiety.

REFERENCES

Abbot, S. K. et al. "Fatty acid composition of membrane bilayers: Importance of diet polyunsaturated fat balance." Biochim Biophys Acta. 2012 May;1818(5):1309-17. doi: 10.1016/j.bbamem.2012.01.011. Epub 2012 Jan 18. PMID: 22285120

Angoa-Perez, M. et al. "Mice Genetically Depleted of Brain Serotonin Do Not Display a Depression-like Behavioral Phenotype." *ACS Chem. Neurosci.*, 2014, 5 (10), pp 908–919

Babu, A.S. et al. "Virgin coconut oil and its potential cardioprotective effects." Postgrad Med. 2014 Nov;126(7):76-83. doi: 10.3810/pgm.2014.11.2835. PMID:25387216

"Bad Bug Book Foodborne Pathogenic Microorganisms and Natural Toxins Handbook Phytohaemagglutinin." United States Food and Drug Administration. Silver Spring, MD. 2013.

Bartolotta, S. et al. "Effect of fatty acids on arenavirus replication: inhibition of virus production by lauric acid." Arch Virol. 2001;146(4):777-90. PMID:11402863

Brown, M. and Goldstein, J. *Nobel Lectures.* Stockholm, Sweden. The Nobel Foundation. 1985.

Carvalho Pereira, D. et al. "Association between obesity and calcium:phosphorus ratio in the habitual diets of adults in a city of Northeastern Brazil: an epidemiological study." Nutr J. 2013; 12: 90. PMCID: PMC3702524

Chek, Paul. CHEK Practitioner and Holistic Lifestyle Coach Programs. San Diego, CA: CHEK Institute, 2001-2012.

Clark, S.D. and Hembree, J. "Inhibition of triiodothyronine's induction of rat liver lipogenic enzymes by dietary fat." J Nutr. 1990 Jun;120(6):625-30. PMID: 2352037

Crane, J.D. et al. "Inhibiting peripheral serotonin synthesis reduces obesity and metabolic dysfunction by promoting brown adipose tissue thermogenesis." Nat Med. 2015 Feb;21(2):166-72. doi: 10.1038/nm.3766. PMID: 25485911

Dayrit, Conrado. "Coconut Oil in Health and Disease: Its and Monolaurin's Potential as a Cure for HIV/AIDS." *XXXVII Cocotech Meeting.* Chennai, India: 2000.

"Eating Fish for Heart Health." American Heart Association. Dallas, TX.

Fallon, S. and Enig, M. "Tragedy and Hype: Third International Soy Symposium."

The Weston A. Price Foundation for Wise Traditions in Food, Farming, and the Healing Arts. Washington, DC. 2000.

Fasano, A. et al. "Prevalence of celiac disease in at-risk and not-at-risk groups in the United States: a large multicenter study." Arch Intern Med. 2003 Feb 10;163(3):286-92. PMID:12578508

Gandotra, S. et al. "Efficacy of Adjunctive Extra Virgin Coconut Oil Use in Moderate to Severe Alzheimer's Disease." *International Journal of School and Cognitive Psychology.*

Genuis, S.A. and Lobo, R.A. "Gluten sensitivity presenting as a neuropsychiatric disorder. Gastroenterol Res Pract. 2014;2014:293206. PMID:24693281

Guyton, Arthur and Hall, John. The Textbook of Medical Physiology. Philadelphia, PA: Saunders, 2000.

Hayat, Mathew J. et al. "Cancer Statistics, Trends, and Multiple Primary Cancer Analyses from the Surveillance, Epidemiology, and End Results (SEER) Program." *The Oncologist.* 2006.

Hayatullina, Z. et al. "Virgin coconut oil supplementation prevents bone loss in osteoporosis rat model." Evid Based Complement Alternat Med. 2012;2012:237236. PMID:23024690

Jackson, J.R. et al. "Neurologic and psychiatric manifestations of celiac disease and gluten sensitivity." Psychiatr Q. 2012 Mar;83(1):91-102. PMID:21877216

Jenkins, D. et al. Glycemic index of foods: a physiological basis for carbohydrate exchange. *The American Journal of Clinical Nutrition.* 1981.

Johnson, I.T. et al. "Influence of saponins on gut permeability and active nutrient transport in vitro." J Nutr. 1986 Nov;116(11):2270-7. PMID:3794833

Kalaydjian, A.E. et al. "The gluten connection: the association between schizophrenia and celiac disease." Acta Psychiatr Scand. 2006 Feb;113(2):82-90. PMID:16423158

Kemi, V.E. et al. "Increased calcium intake does not completely counteract the effects of increased phosphorus intake on bone: an acute dose-response study in healthy females." Br J Nutr. 2008 Apr;99(4):832-9. PMID:17903344

Keys, Ancel. The Seven Countries Study.

Klandorf, H. et al. "Effect of fatty acid administration on plasma thyroid hormones in the domestic fowl." Gen Comp Endocrinol. 1988 Jun;70(3):395-400. PMID: 3417114

"Known and Probably Human Carcinogens." American Cancer Society. Atlanta, GA, 2015.

Lattimer, J. and Haub, M. "Effects of Dietary Fiber and Its Components on Metabolic Health." *Nutrients.* 2010 Dec; 2(12): 1266–1289. PMCID: PMC3257631

Marieb, Elaine N. Human Anatomy and Physiology. Redwood City, CA: The Benjamin/Cummings Publishing Company, 1992.

Moffett, John R. and Namboodiri, Aryan. "Tryptophan and the immune response." *Immunology and Cell Biology.* 2003.

Moncrieff, J. and Cohen, D. "Do Antidepressants Cure or Create Abnormal Brain States?" PLoS Med. 2006 Jul; 3(7): e240. PMCID: PMC1472553

Montgomery, M.K. et al. "Contrasting metabolic effects of medium- versus long-chain fatty acids in skeletal muscle." *Journal of Lipid Research.* 2013 Dec;54(12):3322-33. doi: 10.1194/jlr.M040451. PMID:24078708

Nakatsuji, T. et al. "Antimicrobial property of lauric acid against Propionibacterium acnes: its therapeutic potential for inflammatory acne vulgaris." J Invest Dermatol. 2009 Oct;129(10):2480-8. doi: 10.1038/jid.2009.93. Epub 2009 Apr 23. PMID:19387482

Oqbolu, D.O. et al. "In vitro antimicrobial properties of coconut oil on Candida species in Ibadan, Nigeria." J Med Food. 2007 Jun;10(2):384-7. PMID:17651080

"Overweight and Obesity." Centers for Disease Control and Prevention. Atlanta, GA.

Piovesan, D. et al. 3,751 magnesium binding sites have been detected on human proteins. *BMC Bioinformatics.* 2012 ;13 Suppl 14:S10. Epub 2012 Sep 7. PMID: 23095498

Price, Weston A. Nutrition and Physical Degeneration. La Mesa, CA: The Price-Pottenger Nutrition Foundation, 2004.

Reger, M.A. et al. "Effects of beta-hydroxybutyrate on cognition in memory-impaired adults." Neurobiol Aging. 2004 Mar;25(3):311-4. PMID:15123336

Robinson, Byron. The Abdominal and Pelvic Brain. Charleston, SC: Nabu Press, 2010.

Samsel, A. and Seneff, S. "Glyphosate, pathways to modern diseases II: Celiac Sprue and Gluten Intolerance." *Interdisciplinary Toxicology.* 2013.

Schmidt, R. et al. "Altered fatty acid composition of lung surfactant phospholipids in interstitial lung disease." Am J Physiol Lung Cell Mol Physiol. 2002 Nov;283(5):L1079-85. PMID: 12376361

Scudellari, M. "Power Failure." *The Scientist.* 2011.

Singh, M. "Wheat gluten as a pathogenic factor in schizophrenia." Science. 1976 Jan 30;191(4225):401-2.

"Soybean Promotion and Research Program Background Information." United States Department of Agriculture. 2014.

Story, John and Klurfeld, David. "David Kritchevsky". *The Journal of Nutrition.* 2007.

Sowers, J.R. et al. "Narrative review: the emerging clinical implications of the role of aldosterone in the metabolic syndrome and resistant hypertension." Ann Intern Med. 2009 Jun 2;150(11):776-83. PMID:19487712

Steiber, A. and Tuma, P. "Academy Comments re The DGAC Scientific Report." Academy of Nutrition and Dietetics. 2015.

Tobacman, J.K. "Review of harmful gastrointestinal effects of carrageenan in animal experiments." Environ Health Perspect. 2001 Oct; 109(10): 983–994. PMCID: PMC1242073

Vysakh, A. et al. "Polyphenolics isolated from virgin coconut oil inhibits adjuvant induced arthritis in rats through antioxidant and anti-inflammatory action." Int Immunopharmacol. 2014 May;20(1):124-30. doi: 10.1016/j.intimp.2014.02.026. PMID: 24613207

Watkins, B A, and M F Seifert, "Food Lipids and Bone Health," *Food Lipids and Health.* New York, NY: Marcel Dekker, Inc, 1996

Zakariah, Z.A. et al. "Hepatoprotective Activity of Dried- and Fermented-Processed Virgin Coconut Oil." Evidence-Based Complementary and Alternative Medicine Volume 2011 (2011), Article ID 142739

RESOURCES

- **http://www.alterecofoods.com/products/chocolate/** You know what kind of man you're dealing with when he puts a link to chocolate first in the Resources section of his book. But chocolate is a good source of nutrition—from magnesium to saturated fat—and a staple in my diet. Most sources will be loaded with soy lecithin or other junk. This brand is clean, and you will taste the difference.
- **http://www.chekinstitute.com/** Where my education began and where it will truly never end. Paul Chek's *Holistic Lifestyle Level 1* is where I would start if I was embarking on the road to health all over again. But there are plenty of other learning opportunities offered here for those brave enough to take responsibility for themselves.
- **http://www.ewg.org/** If it's on your skin, it's in your body. This site empowers you with information via an extensive database (**http://www.ewg.org/skindeep/**), so you can choose your personal care products wisely, minimizing your exposure to xenoestrogens and other carcinogenic chemicals.
- **https://georgiaorganics.org/for-eaters/** The source for all things organic for my local Georgia readers. And I'm sure you can find your state's site with a quick internet search.
- **http://www.greatlakesgelatin.com/** I wish I got a commission from these guys, because I've referred hundreds of people to them. There aren't many supplements I recommend or use personally. But the health benefits of balancing one's amino acid profile put their hydrolyzed and non-hydrolyzed gelatin high on my list. And for those not willing to make their own bone broth, I believe Great Lakes Gelatin to be essential.
- **http://www.localharvest.org/** If you believe in thinking globally by acting locally, this site is for you. Find organic farmers, grocers, and community supported agriculture wherever you may be located in the United States.
- **http://www.nongmoproject.org/** The fight against GMOs is far from over. And unless more people become informed and take action, our health and the health of our environment are in grave danger. This site is a good resource if you want to get involved, and I hope you do.
- **http://www.organic.org/** For everything organic—find out why, how, and who so you can make decisions to support your health, the health of your family, and even the health of our world.
- **http://raypeat.com/** Some incredibly deep information regarding proper nutrition and a multitude of other subjects related to health. Be forewarned, however—it's not easy reading!
- **http://www.realmilk.com/** It takes life to give life. Pasteurized means dead. Take advantage of the many health benefits of raw dairy (including being able to consume it again for those who may be sensitive) by using this site to find a source near you.
- **https://www.theochocolate.com/our-product-info** Yes, another chocolate source!
- **http://triumphtraining.com/** My website and, perhaps, a shameless plug.

- **http://triumphtraining.com/blogs/blog** My blog has been neglected of late because of this project, but it's still rather extensive. The quality of the information you'll find there is inversely proportional to how mainstream it is. So feel free to help yourself so you will be better prepared to help yourself.
- **http://triumphtraining.com/pages/holistic-strength-training-for-triathlon** Immediately download my first book or, if you're more of a traditionalist, get a physical copy. Either way, don't let the title fool you. The book is really a primer on how to train. Triathletes were simply my target audience (as they need a lot of help). But the information within these pages is applicable to anyone interested in health and fitness.
- **http://triumphtraining.com/pages/recommendations** A number of books and other products and services are listed here—and not simply because I recommend them. I use them myself.
- **http://www.westonaprice.org/** An excellent site for those who believe that Mother Nature isn't stupid; and anytime Man tries to improve her, we typically screw things up.

Bone Broth/Gelatin Recipe

Ingredients:

5-6 pounds bones and connective tissue (any type will work, but chicken feet and oxtail make the best broth in my experience)

2 Tablespoons apple-cider vinegar (to help leach minerals out of the bones)

5-6 quarts filtered water (1 qt per lb animal parts)

Potatoes and carrots, chopped, if desired (I don't use any)

Instructions:

1. Place animal parts in large crock pot. Cover with water.
2. Add apple-cider vinegar and/or veggies if desired.
3. Cover and cook for at least 5-6 hours.
4. Remove bones and other large parts. Then strain into a separate glass container(s).
5. Place strained broth in refrigerator until fat has risen to top (usually about 24 hours).
6. Remove fat from top of gelatin, and keep the gelatin refrigerated between uses.

The gelatin should be similar in consistency to Jell-O. If it's more watery, you may have used too much water or gelatin-poor bones. Gelatin can be placed in smoothies or yogurts or sauces without being noticeable. If you enjoy the flavor and tradition, you can heat the gelatin so it returns to a broth and drink it like tea. Either way, the health benefits are enormous.

Broth should keep in the refrigerator for up to a week. Freeze when making bigger batches or when storing longer. Just make sure to fill the glass container(s) only part way as the broth will expand as it freezes.

Carrot Salad Recipe (I originally got this recipe from Dodie Anderson, but modified it a bit to suit my lack of culinary skills)

Ingredients:

1 medium carrot (or equivalent), washed, unpeeled, and grated lengthwise (grating the carrot lengthwise maximizes the toxin-binding effects of the carrot's fibers.)

A drizzling of coconut oil, melted or olive oil (Coconut oil is the better choice as it balances the unsaturated fats, reducing their toxicity. Additionally, it helps heal the intestinal wall and keeps bacterial growth in check.)

Pickling or sea salt to taste (lowers adrenalin, aldosterone, and serotonin while helping to maintain blood sugar and optimal hydration levels.)

A splash of Vinegar (antimicrobial and stimulates the production of Hydrochloric Acid.)

Instructions:

1. Mix
2. Eat

Consumed with a meal, hypoglycemia can result as the absorption of some nutrients from other foods will be slowed. Thus, I recommend eating the carrot/carrot salad on an empty stomach.

A carrot salad daily is an excellent aid in the body's process of detoxification. The fibers are unique in that they don't feed pathogenic bacteria. They also bind and eliminate estrogen while minimizing cortisol production secondary to lowering serotonin and histamine. This helps up-regulate the thyroid which, of course, improves health. The effects of the fibers are enhanced if grated lengthwise. But half the time, I skip all the prep and just eat the carrot. Bamboo shoots purportedly have the same effect and are better tolerated by some who may suffer from compromised digestion. However, I've never used them, so I cannot speak to their efficacy.

> **NOTE**: *poor liver function (which is common) can impact one's ability to convert carotene into Vitamin A. Thus, if you find the calluses on your hands turning orange after using this recipe everyday, I recommend rinsing the grated carrot and squeezing out any orange-colored juice before dressing with coconut/ olive oil and salt as described in the above recipe.*

Cooked Apple Recipe

Ingredients:

Apples
Brown Sugar
Butter
Cinnamon
Coconut Oil
Great Lakes Gelatin

Instructions:

You'll notice I didn't include any amounts in the ingredients listed above. Maybe my left/logical brain could use some stimulus, but I typically just go by taste. I use 3-5 apples, depending on the size of the apples, the size of the bowl in which I'm cooking, and the size of my appetite. I then add some coconut oil, a generous supply of butter, more brown sugar than some might think is healthy, and a few solid shakes of cinnamon. Once it gets soupy, I add the gelatin and any of the aforementioned ingredients I think is missing in sufficient amounts. Then I let it cook until the apples are at the desired level of firmness—soft but with a hint of crispness still. Eaten warm, it's like apple pie filling. But if I put it in the fridge to congeal, I can then cut them up into incredibly satisfying apple-gel blocks for training or snacks. In fact, those blocks are what has fueled me to my Half-Ironman PR (4:11) as well as my win in the Great Floridian—both at the age of forty.

Eggshell Calcium Recipe
Ingredients:
Eggshells
Instructions:

1. Wash empty eggshells in warm water until all of the egg white is removed (take care not to remove the membrane—it contains other nutrients in addition to calcium).
2. Lay broken pieces on paper towels, allowing them to air dry thoroughly.
3. Break the eggshells up into small pieces (a coffee grinder works best) until they are the consistency of a powder. Store powder in a glass container.

1/2 teaspoon equals approximately 400mg of calcium carbonate along with a good quantity of other micronutrients. Mixed in foods, you may find it a bit gritty. Taken by the spoonful and chased with water is the most practical method of supplementing.

Smoothie Recipe
Ingredients:
Frozen fruit (I don't believe apples, pears, or melons work well, but any other is fine)
Milk
Gelatin/Bone Broth
Raw Cocoa Powder
Refined Coconut Oil
Salt
Honey (if necessary)
Instructions:

Put in all in a blender and push the button. Seriously, I don't measure any of the ingredients. The fruit is usually enough to fill the blender half-way. I then pour milk until the fruit is mostly submerged. Next I put in several spoonfuls of bone broth and pour a generous portion of Great Lakes Gelatin on top. I add a heaping tablespoon of coconut oil, 3-4 tablespoons of cocoa, and then several shakes of salt. If necessary (and it usually is if I'm making a raspberry smoothie for my wife), I use honey to taste. Blend, eat, and try your best to share if your spouse is around.

ABOUT THE AUTHOR

A native of Atlanta, Andrew Johnston has been involved in personal training for over fifteen years. He originally got into the business for self-improvement, arming himself with knowledge to combat the performance-enhancing drugs that inundate the sport of professional cycling. The strategy worked, and in 1992 he was invited to be a resident athlete at the Olympic Training Center in Colorado Springs. Upon graduation from Eckerd College in 1994, he turned pro and took his ambitions to Europe to race for the Belgian Haverbeke GB team. After the 1996 Olympic Trials, he moved to Spain to race for the Palafrugell and Homs squads until 1998. Andrew devoted his full attention to personal training in 1999, after a crash ended his cycling career just as he was entering his prime. But his competitive juices were quenched for only a year before he discovered an interest in triathlon. In his first full season of triathlon competition, he was the 2001 Olympic Distance Champion of Georgia and fifth overall at the National Long Course Triathlon Championships, earning All-American status as well as a slot on the US World Triathlon team.

Andrew founded Triumph Training in 2000, turning his athletic experience and insatiable appetite for knowledge into a successful athletic and rehabilitation training business. Not content with having obtained his Certified Strength and Conditioning Specialist degree, arguably the most respected credential in the fitness industry, Andrew became the first Corrective Holistic Exercise Kinesiologist in the state of Georgia in 2001. His passion for the body and its limitless potential has since grown only stronger, with *Men's Journal* naming him one of the *"Top 100 Trainers in the US"* two years in a row. By practicing what he preaches to his clientele as well as various audiences throughout the Southeast, Andrew became the first Leukemia Survivor to qualify for and finish the Hawaii Ironman World Championships in 2006. The award-winning documentary *Living is Winning* captures the events leading up to that race and takes the audience deep into the life of an aspiring triathlete. He followed up that feat by becoming the first Leukemia Survivor to win the Overall of an Iron Distance Triathlon as the 2012 Champion of the Great Floridian Triathlon. Now Andrew uses his knowledge as a Holistic Lifestyle Coach and CHEK practitioner to guide people in their pursuit of wellness, ultimately helping them to realize that the only limitations they truly have are the ones they impose on themselves.

For more information on coaching, training, or speaking, Andrew Johnston can be reached by e-mail at **Andrew@triumphtraining.com**.

Made in the USA
Columbia, SC
25 June 2020